PHYSICAL EXERCISE, NUTRITION AND STRESS

PHYSICAL EXERCISE, NUTRITION AND STRESS

Mary F. Asterita, Ph.D.

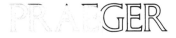

PRAEGER

PRAEGER SPECIAL STUDIES • PRAEGER SCIENTIFIC

New York • Philadelphia • Eastbourne, UK
Toronto • Hong Kong • Tokyo • Sydney

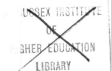

Published and Distributed by the
Praeger Publishers Division
(ISBN Prefix 0-275)
of Greenwood Press, Inc.,
Westport, Connecticut

Library of Congress Cataloging-in-Publication Data

Asterita, Mary F. (Mary Frances)
  Physical exercise, nutrition and stress.

  Bibliography: p.
  Includes index.
  1. Exercise--Physiological aspects.
2. Exercise--Nutritional aspects.   3. Stress
(Physiology)   I. Title.
QP303.A77   1985   612'.76   85-12261
ISBN 0-03-000468-3 (alk. paper)

Published in 1986 by Praeger Publishers
CBS Educational and Professional Publishing, a Division of CBS Inc.
521 Fifth Avenue, New York, NY 10175 USA

Printed in the United States of America on acid-free paper

INTERNATIONAL OFFICES

Orders from outside the United States should be sent to the appropriate address listed below. Orders from areas not
listed below should be placed through CBS International Publishing, 383 Madison Ave., New York, NY 10175 USA

Australia, New Zealand
Holt Saunders, Pty, Ltd., 9 Waltham St., Artarmon, N.S.W. 2064, Sydney, Australia

Canada
Holt, Rinehart & Winston of Canada, 55 Horner Ave., Toronto, Ontario, Canada M8Z 4X6

Europe, the Middle East, & Africa
Holt Saunders, Ltd., 1 St. Anne's Road, Eastbourne, East Sussex, England BN21 3UN

Japan.
Holt Saunders, Ltd., Ichibancho Central Building, 22-1 Ichibancho, 3rd Floor, Chiyodaku, Tokyo, Japan

Hong Kong, Southeast Asia
Holt Saunders Asia, Ltd., 10 Fl, Intercontinental Plaza, 94 Granville Road, Tsim Sha Tsui East, Kowloon,
Hong Kong

**Manuscript submissions should be sent to the Editorial Director, Praeger Publishers, 521 Fifth Avenue,
New York, NY 10175 USA**

DEDICATED TO

*My dear Aunt Dolly and Aunt Tessie, who, through the
strength and fortitude they have shown in their lives,
have touched the hearts of many, with esteem and inspiration.*

PREFACE

In recent years, the psychophysiological components of stress and their relation to human health and disease have been the focus of much attention and have been the subject of several scientific investigative efforts throughout many countries of the world. Stress has been studied from many avenues of approach, including the psychological (mental and emotional), behavioral, and physiological points of view. Many studies are also available that describe stress in terms of its relationship to lifestyle, management, and treatment. All of these studies taken together contribute toward a comprehensive treatment and understanding of stress and its influence on the state of health of the organism.

This book is an attempt to isolate two important areas of physiology—exercise and nutrition—and to investigate the effects of exercise stress on the physical body and the effects of stress on the nutritional status of the organism. The purpose of this book is therefore twofold. First, it aims to briefly describe the major physiological changes that take place in the human body as a result of the stress of physical exercise. Secondly, it discusses in brief and general terms the various nutrients important to the proper physiological functioning of the body and the effects of various types of stress exposure on these nutrients. The material presented in this text discusses the stress response from a general scientific point of view based on current scientific knowledge and research findings.

This book is intended to be used as a general source guide for health care professionals—including practicing clinicians, physicians, psychologists, nutritionists, exercise physiologists, physical and behavioral therapists, nurses and others—who daily deal with clients experiencing psychophysiological stress arousal states.

While this book makes no claims to be all-inclusive with regard to a description of the physiological effects of the stress of physical exercise and of the effects of stress on the various nutrients described, it is the aim of this text to present the current facts known, so that a generalized knowledge of the subject may be gained. In addition, the effects of stress on the various nutrients are described in terms of some of the scientific research reported in the literature within the last few decades. The scientific research work described does not include all the scientific research available to date, but is merely representative of other similar and notable published research. It is not the intent of this book to single out any one scientific research work as more meritorious than another, but simply to present a limited review of the scientific literature so that the reader can gain a greater comprehension and appreciation for the work involved in advancing scientific knowledge in the field of physical exercise and nutrition stress. In addition, this book makes no claims to being a final, definitive work in this field but does aim to update and bring together important knowledge and key areas of research regarding the stress of physical exercise and the effects of stress on the various nutrients found in the body.

Mary F. Asterita, Ph.D.

ACKNOWLEDGMENTS

This book was made possible because of the help and support of many of my colleagues and friends. The following individuals deserve much thanks for contributing their time and efforts in making this book become a reality: to Dr. Charles Stroebel, Dr. Donald Macchia, and Dr. Richard Malter, who have contributed much of their time to review the manuscript and offer their professional insight; to Dr. Richard Malter, who has also contributed his time and professional assistance in writing the section on hair analysis in Chapter 7; to Donya Warren and Rose Marie Ward for contributing their time and talents and word processor skills to produce this manuscript in its final form; and to all others at the Northwest Center for Medical Education, Indiana University School of Medicine, who have contributed their support and professional assistance. Finally, special thanks goes to my mother and father, my brothers Tony and Joseph and their families, and my many friends for their continuing kindness, understanding, and loving support.

CONTENTS

PHYSICAL EXERCISE,
NUTRITION
AND STRESS

1

INTRODUCTION

STRESS: DEFINITION

The study of stress in its many facets has gained much momentum in the last few decades. Stress is now recognized as an important factor related to several disorders and disease states prevalent in society today. Stress was first described by Selye (1950, 1957, 1976) and is associated with a mental/emotional/physical state produced within an organism in response to a stimulus (whether internal or external) that is perceived as a threat (stressor). There are many ways to define and discuss stress without going into a lengthy philosophical discussion. A rather general definition is included here and is sufficient to suit our purposes.

Stress can be described as a wide range of physiological and biochemical changes that take place in the physical body, either in acute or chronic conditions, that are induced by various psychological (mental and emotional) or physical factors (stimuli) or a combination of these factors, and that are perceived by the organism as a threat. The experience of stress induces a stress response, which is a specific response characterized by various psychological, physiological, and behavioral components. It is a state of psychophysiological arousal within the organism and initiates the activation of neural, neuroendocrine, endocrine, biochemical, metabolic and other components, all of which constitute the specific physiological characteristics of the stress response itself.

TYPES OF STRESS

Whenever the organism perceives a stimulus as a threat, whether internal or external, the stimulus is referred to as a stressor. Stressors may be physical or psychological.

Types of physical stressors include such conditions as crowding, isolation, extreme changes in temperature, and the presence of chemical pollutants or toxic mineral elements in the environment or in the physical body. Physical stressors may also be physiological in nature, such as states of hypoglycemia, shock, trauma, infection, pain, or prolonged exercise.

Psychological stress or psychogenically induced stress can result from one's own mental and emotional reactivity patterns to one's own inner cognitions and emotions or to outside influences such as persons, places, and events in one's environment.

While the stress response itself is characterized by an array of biochemical and physiological changes in the physical body, this response may be elicited in varying degrees in different individuals confronting the same stressor. A stimulus that may induce the stress response or, in other words, be stressful for one individual may or may not be a source of stress for another individual. Also, what may act as a stressor for one individual at one particular time may or may not act as a stressor for the same individual at a later time. The stressor can assume many forms and the resulting stress response can arise from a variety of causes. In examining the short- or long-term physiological effects of the stress response, several important factors should therefore be kept in mind. Also, the effects of the stress response should always be viewed in terms of the individual variations in perception, the intensity of individual reactivity to the stressor, and the chronicity of the stressor.

THE STRESS RESPONSE

The physical body responds to stimuli perceived as a threat in a very specific manner. The response by the body, termed the stress response, consists of a biochemically regulated set of physiological changes that govern several organ systems and chemical reactions in the body. The physiological changes that take place as a result of the stress response are an effort by the organism to achieve physiological balance and adaptation in situations of chronic stress. These physiological changes contribute toward the reestablishment and maintenance of normal metabolism and homeostasis.

The physiology of the stress response has been clearly described in several texts dealing with the subject (Asterita 1985; Everly, Jr. and Rosenfeld 1981). A brief description is presented here for review.

Basically, the stress response is associated with an activation of a neural and several neuroendocrine pathways in the body. The primary neural response results in an activation of the sympathetic portion of the autonomic nervous system. This in turn results in several physiological responses associated with sympathetic arousal. This enhancement of sympathetic activity triggers the well-known neuroendocrine "fight or flight" response, which involves sympathetic stimulation of the adrenal medulla, which, in turn, results in the hormonal output of epinephrine and norepinephrine by the adrenal gland. These hormones intensify the sympathetic response, some of which includes an increase in heart rate and blood pressure, pupillary dilatation, a shunting of the blood away from the periphery and into the muscular system, an increase in muscle tone, dry mouth, an increase in sweat gland activity, and a shallower and increased rate of respiration. These physiological changes are the underlying factors involved in the experience of increased anxiety and tension associated with the elicitation of the stress response.

The stress response in its more chronic phase involves further stimulation of the neuroendocrine axis, which, in turn, involves the stimulation or inhibition of secretion of several hormones into the circulation. The presence of these hormones initiates several physiological and biochemical changes that aid the organism in adaptation to the stressor. Involved in practically all types of stress exposures is the increase in adrenal cortical hormone secretion, mediated by the hypothalamo-anterior pituitary-adrenal cortical axis. Adrenocorticotropin-releasing hormone from the hypothalamus stimulates the release of adrenocorticotropin hormone (ACTH) by the anterior pituitary, which is carried in the circulation to the adrenal cortex and stimulates this gland to release the hormone cortisol. The release of cortisol into the circulation as a result of the stress response serves many important functions. Some of these functions relate to changes in metabolism:

- a stimulation of protein breakdown (protein catabolism).
- a stimulation of amino acid (the product of protein breakdown) uptake by the liver. The amino acid uptake by the liver enhances liver gluconeogenesis, which is the production of glucose from noncarbohydrate sources. In this case, the amino acids provide an added source of energy for the body, and any amino acids that are released into the circulation become available for tissue repair in the face of any tissue trauma or damage that may occur as a result of stress exposure.

- a permissive effect for the stimulation of gluconeogenesis by other stress hormones.
- a stimulation of hypergylcemia with a decrease in glucose uptake by many cells of the body, excluding the brain and muscle cells. Hence there is an abundant source of energy available, in the form of glucose, for the brain and muscle cells.
- a stimulation of the use of fats for energy. The glucose utilization by many cells of the body is therefore replaced by the presence of free fatty acids (FFA) that have been released from adipose tissue. Free fatty acids act as a source of energy in place of glucose.

In summary, stress-induced cortisol secretion promotes protein and fat mobilization and gluconeogenesis. These metabolic effects of cortisol provide the organism with the necessary fuel and energy to meet the stressful encounter adequately and efficiently.

Because of the presence of the hormones epinephrine, norepinephrine, and cortisol in the circulation as a result of the stress response, greater sources of energy are mobilized, and the vital organs such as the brain, heart, and muscles are provided with plenty of nutrients (glucose) and fuel at the expense of other tissues such as the skin and gastrointestinal tract.

In the more chronic phase of the stress response, other endocrine axes are activated, leading to the secretion of several other hormones into the circulation. The elevated blood glucose levels lead to increases in pancreatic glucagon secretion. This hormone stimulates liver glycogenolysis, which adds more glucose into the circulation. In many instances, insulin secretion is depressed. Other hormones that are usually released as a result of stress include aldosterone and antidiuretic hormone (ADH). These two hormones enhance the retention of sodium and water by the body, which can be an important adaptive response. Another hormone generally secreted as a result of stress is growth hormone. In concert with glucagon, it enhances blood glucose levels and stimulates the uptake of amino acids by cells, in particular the cells of injured tissue, so that tissue repair can more easily take place if needed.

Other hormones influenced by stress include the pituitary gonadotropins, leutinizing hormone (LH), and follicle-stimulating hormone (FSH), which regulate the secretion of the sex hormones (estrogen and progesterone in the female and testosterone in the male). LH, FSH, and the sex hormones, like insulin, are depressed as a result of the stress response. In the female, the monthly cycle of hormonal secretions involving FSH, LH, estrogen, and progesterone can be altered as a result of stress and therefore changed from its normal cyclic pattern. In many types of stress exposure, the thyroid hormones also appear to be suppressed.

Other hormones whose secretions are known to be stimulated as a result of the stress response include the endogenous opiates and prolactin. The physiological mechanisms and significance involved in the enhanced levels of these hormones in the circulation as a result of the stress response remains to be elucidated. Also, the adaptive significance of many of these hormonal changes, while not definitively clarified, may play an important role in the various known stress-induced disease states.

The more chronic neuroendocrine phase of the stress response involves a large measure of variability. Many of the hormones may or may not be stimulated, but when they are, it is with different degrees of intensity and chronicity. During chronic stress, the type, severity, and chronicity of the stress exposure, along with the degree of intensity with which the stress exposure is perceived and is experienced, contribute to the nature of the total neuroendocrine response pattern.

The next chapter discusses the stress of physical exercise. The physiological changes that occur in the different systems of the body as well as the hormonal changes that occur as a result of the stress of physical exercise are briefly described.

2

PHYSICAL EXERCISE

The stress of physical exercise involves a change in several biochemical and physiological processes in the body. It is well known that exercise has profound effects on the various systems of the body, depending on how strenuous the exercise is. Exercise also enhances the rate of metabolism and can influence the concentration of certain metabolites and hormones in the circulation. The following discussion provides a brief survey of the physiological changes that take place in the various systems of the body, including the major hormonal changes that occur in response to the stress of physical exercise.

BODY TEMPERATURE

During prolonged exercise, the metabolic rate increases approximately 10 to 20 times above normal. Approximately 80 percent of the total amount of energy consumed in the body during exercise is in the form of thermal energy or heat from the increase in metabolism. The other 20 percent of energy used comes from the contraction of muscles. Therefore, the increase in body temperature that occurs during exercise is directly related to the heat produced from metabolic activity and is not a function of the ambient environmental temperature. Also, the significance of the rise in body temperature in exercise performance is not entirely clear. Warmup exercises increase blood flow to the muscles, which provides thermal energy to enhance muscle cell metabolism. The transfer of oxygen from the blood to the tissues is also increased, thereby rendering the respiratory diffusion of oxygen and carbon dioxide more effective and efficient.

RESPIRATORY SYSTEM

Because of the increase in cellular metabolism (oxygen consumption and carbon dioxide production) during exercise, the respiratory system functions with much greater capacity. The total work of breathing may increase 100 times above normal. Additional muscles are recruited into use in order to participate in the whole process of the mechanics of breathing. Pulmonary ventilation may reach as high as 150 liters per minute, increasing from a normal baseline level of approximately 5 or 6 liters per minute. This change results from an increase in the rate of breathing from about 15 to 40 or 50 breaths per minute and an increase in tidal volume of about a few liters above normal levels. Because of these changes, the lungs, during exercise, absorb a great amount of oxygen, much more than normal, sometimes ranging up to 20 times the ordinary amount. For all individuals, under normal conditions, basal oxygen consumption is approximately 250 milliliters (ml) per minute. An untrained athlete can increase oxygen consumption approximately 3 times normal during light exercise. A trained athlete can increase this amount up to 20 times normal (about 4 to 5 liters per minute). The change in oxygen consumption depends on how strenuous the exercise is. The lungs have therefore a very great capacity to absorb very large amounts of oxygen during strenuous exercise.

Because of the increase in cardiac output (the amount of blood pumped by the heart each minute), blood flow to the lungs is increased. Several pulmonary capillary beds also open up, which contributes to the increase of blood flow to the lungs. This increase in blood flow facilitates the exchange of oxygen and carbon dioxide. The blood volume of the lungs can increase from approximately 60 to 90 ml in untrained individuals and from approximately 70 to 200 ml for the trained athlete. The increase in blood volume occurs without any significant increase in pulmonary arterial pressure and therefore helps in the prevention of pulmonary edema during the elevated cardiac output. While a greater amount of oxygen and carbon dioxide is handled by the lungs during exercise, the oxygen and carbon dioxide tensions of the blood change only slightly and essentially remain within normal limits, thereby minimizing any pH changes. Also, even though large amounts of muscle lactic acid are produced (only in severely strenuous exercise), several regulatory mechanisms come into play to maintain the acid-base status within normal limits.

CIRCULATION

During exercise, many capillary beds which are distributed through-out the skeletal muscular system that are closed under normal conditions, open up during exercise. This greatly enhances blood flow to the skeletal muscles. The increase in mean arterial pressure that occurs, accompanied by an increase in cardiac output, also contributes to the enhanced blood flow through muscle capillaries. In addition, there is a dramatic increase in blood flow to the respiratory muscles, heart, and skin. The blood flow to the brain and the kidneys is generally maintained as under normal conditions, but splanchnic blood flow is decreased. Several regulatory mechanisms come into play to allow for the adjustments in blood flow to the various organs and systems. These mechanisms include the activity of the sympathetic nervous system, the endocrine hormonal secretions, autoregulation, and the presence of local metabolites. All of these factors interact in a particular way to allow for the observed physiological adjustments that take place in blood flow during exercise.

CARDIOVASCULAR SYSTEM

The most profound effects of exercise are seen in the cardiovascular system. The strength of the heart increases and the effectiveness of the heart as a pump likewise increases. During exercise, large quantities of venous blood are returned to the heart from the peripheral systemic circulation and from the muscular system. The vasodilation that occurs in the arterioles of the muscular system during exercise contributes to the elevation in cardiac output of about four or even seven times normal, which equates to about 20 to 35 liters per minute, again, depending on how strenuous the exercise is. Cardiac output may therefore increase from a resting or normal value of 5 liters per minute to values as high as 35 liters per minute. The increase in cardiac output is also proportional to the increase in oxygen consumption that takes place during exercise. This increase in cardiac output provides the necessary increased amounts of oxygen, nutrients, and hormones to be transported to the various tissues of the body and transport of carbon dioxide away from the tissues needed during this time of stress.

To achieve the high increase in cardiac output, several factors must come into play. For one thing, the sympathetic nervous system is activated. The sympathetic vasodilator fibers to the skeletal muscles provide the increase in blood flow to these muscles. This is especially true in strenuous exercise and need not be the case in lighter exercise. While a sympathetic mediated increase in blood flow occurs in the skeletal muscles during strenuous or intense exercise, a simultaneous sympathetic stimulation causes a vasoconstriction of most of the blood vessels to other organs of the body, such as the kidneys and gastrointestinal tract. The net result of this is a marked decrease in the total peripheral resistance. In strenuous exercise, sympathetic stimulation of the heart and circulation is necessary, but in lighter exercise, sympathetic activity of the cardiovascular system appears not be as necessary.

Other factors may be involved in stimulation of the sympathetic nervous system during exercise. Reflex stimulation of the sympathetic nervous system may occur by means of contraction of the muscles themselves. Also, the same signals from the motor cortex that stimulate muscle activity may also stimulate the sympathetic nervous system. Signals from the motor cortex may stimulate vasodilator fibers of the sympathetic nervous system that go directly to the skeletal muscles in order to enhance blood flow throughout the muscular system.

At the onset of exercise, the muscles of the abdomen contract, probably because of a generalized increase in muscle tone or tension. This results in a compression of the large venous reservoirs located in the abdominal region, which further contributes to an increase in venous return of blood to the heart. This also contributes to the observed increase in cardiac output.

Other factors that contribute to an increase in cardiac output during exercise are an increase in heart rate (often referred to as a chronotropic effect) and an increase in stroke volume. The heart rate may increase in normal individuals from 75 to 100 beats per minute during light exercise or up to 180 beats per minute in heavy exercise, the upper limit for nonathletes. Both heart rate and stroke volume increase and are associated with a greater increase in cardiac sympathetic activity than parasympathetic activity. The increase in heart rate is usually much greater than the increase that occurs in stroke volume. Stroke volume is simply defined as the amount of blood pumped by the heart per beat. The stroke volume increases from a normal value of about 70 ml per beat in resting males to about 150 ml per beat in exercise. This increase in stroke volume may be a result of the increase in muscular contractility induced by enhanced cardiac sympathetic nerve activity. Also, there is a decrease in the time it takes for cardiac ventricular filling to occur. This is directly related to several factors, among which are the increase in heart rate and an increase in cardiac systemic filling pressure.

The other factor involved in the marked enhancement of cardiac output during physical exercise stress is related to the increased venous return to the heart, caused by (1) a marked increase in respiratory activity, which includes an increase in breathing rate; (2) a great increase in skeletal muscle tone, tension, and blood flow; and (3) the sympathetic mediated enhancement of blood flow from arteries to veins through the dilated blood vessels, the arterioles, of the skeletal muscle system. These factors taken together may provide a rapid and efficient means for the blood in the various vessels of the body to return to the heart and provide for a significant enhancement of cardiac venous return. If venous return

TABLE 2.1. Summary of the Major Physiological Changes Occurring During the Stress of Physical Exercise

Body temperature	increases approximately 2°C.
Metabolic rate:	increases severalfold.
Circulation:	increase in blood flow to the brain, heart, kidneys, lungs, and skeletal muscle; decrease in splanchnic blood flow.
	very little or no changes in acid-base status of the blood.
Respiratory system:	increase in tidal volume, breathing rate, pulmonary ventilation, total work of breathing, diffusion capacity of the lungs for oxygen, oxygen consumption, and carbon dioxide production.
Cardiovascular system:	increase in heart rate, force of contraction of the heart, cardiac output, stroke volume, cardiac systemic filling pressure, systolic arterial pressure, and venous return to the heart.
	no change in end-diastolic volume and diastolic blood pressure.
	decrease in ventricular filling pressure and total peripheral resistance.

is increased in significant amounts, the end-diastolic ventricular volume may increase, which would lead to a further enhancement of stroke volume and cardiac output.

Another important physiological parameter that significantly changes during the stress of physical exercise is the arterial blood pressure. It is a well-known, established fact that the arterial pressure is a function of cardiac output and total peripheral resistance (arterial pressure = cardiac output × total peripheral resistance). As a result of exercise, cardiac output generally increases and total peripheral resistance decreases. Most forms of exercise result in a greater percentage increase in cardiac output than a percentage decrease in total peripheral resistance. The increase in the heart rate causes a more rapid cardiac ejection rate, which generally increases the systolic pressure. Since systolic pressure increases (seldom rising above 180 mmHg in normotensive individuals) while diastolic pressure remains unaffected, the pulse pressure may itself increase proportionately and markedly. The pulse pressure is defined as the difference between the systolic and diastolic pressures. For example, if the systolic pressure is 120 mmHg and the diastolic pressure is 80 mmHg, the difference between the two is equivalent to a pulse pressure of 40 mmHg.

It is interesting to speculate on the mechanisms contributing to the cardiovascular changes that occur during exercise. The interrelationships involved are complex and are not definitely understood. The rise in arterial pressure should influence the arterial baroreceptors to signal the medullary centers to decrease the cardiac output, thus setting up a negative feedback loop that regulates the cardiovascular changes seen in exercise. This obviously does not predominate. The arterial baroreceptors themselves are not the primary cause of the observed cardiovascular changes that take place during exercise since their activity would promote the opposite effects. Perhaps the mechanisms involved relate to the specific center or centers in the hypothalamus that coordinate signals via descending pathways to the medullary centers, which, in turn, produce the pronounced effects in autonomic nervous system activity observed during exercise. The hypothalamus may receive inputs from several other sources within the central nervous system. One possible source would be the signals originating from the motor cortex, as described earlier, which stimulate muscle activity associated with exercise.

Perhaps the same mechanisms and neural inputs involved in the cardiovascular changes during exercise are also involved in the physiological changes that occur during the experience of other types of stress exposures. A summary of the major physiological changes occurring during the stress of physical exercise is presented in Table 2.1.

PSYCHIC STIMULI

The mere process of thinking about exercise can stimulate the centers involved in autonomic nervous system control. By cognitive stimuli, the sympathetic portion of the autonomic nervous system can be activated, which accelerates those familiar processes that lead to an increase in cardiac output. These processes, as mentioned previously, include an increase in heart rate, increase in strength of contraction of the heart, and vasodilation of blood vessels in the skeletal muscular system and throughout other organ systems of the body, which increases both the mean systemic filling pressure and venous return to the heart.

METABOLIC RATE

Exercise also has a profound effect on the metabolic rate of the body, increasing it severalfold, depending on how strenuous the exercise is. In certain instances the metabolic rate can increase to between 1,000 and

2,000 percent of normal. The important metabolic fuels used in exercise are carbohydrates and fats. In light exercise, fats supply most of the required energy. In more strenuous exercise, carbohydrates derived from skeletal muscle glycogen constitute most of the fuel. It appears that in strenuous exercise, the body is able to substitute carbohydrate for lipid but not lipid for carbohydrate. In heavy exercise, when fatigue and exhaustion occur, both appear to be related to a decrease in muscle glycogen or the availability of carbohydrates and glucose.

During exercise, several hormones also come into play to enhance both carbohydrate and fat utilization by the body.

ENDOCRINE SYSTEM

During exercise, the glucose uptake of various tissues of the body balances the glucose output of the liver. All the factors that influence hepatic glucose output are not definitively known but may include neuronal and perhaps hormonal inputs. It is known, however, that the hepatic output of glucose is independent of the presence of insulin and other hormones known to influence blood glucose levels.

Insulin, the catecholamines, epinephrine and norepinephrine, and such hormones as cortisol, growth hormone, and glucagon play a role in the uptake of glucose by several of the body tissues. Exercise-mediated variations in glucose uptake are also affected by changes in the number and binding of insulin receptor sites. Other factors, such as cyclic AMP and any of the rate-limiting enzymes in the glycolytic pathway, may also play a role in influencing tissue glucose uptake (Sutton 1983; Vranic and Berger 1979).

Several mechanisms are involved in the uptake of glucose by muscle cells that have not yet been clearly elucidated. However, it is known that glucose uptake in resting muscle cells is regulated by the presence of insulin. During exercise, it has been observed in many studies, while muscle glucose transport is enhanced, the concentration of insulin itself does not change or, in some cases, may even decrease (Le Blanc et al. 1979; Lohman et al. 1978; Mondon et al. 1980). The regulatory mechanisms involved in this sequence of exercise-induced maintained insulin activity, increase in muscle cell glucose uptake, and muscular contraction, are not clearly defined. Perhaps an enhancement of the insulin-binding capacity to the insulin receptor sites on the muscle membrane is one of the factors involved in the maintained insulin concentration and increase in glucose transport observed during muscle contraction.

Other hormones and factors that influence receptor activity may also play a role in the enhancement of exercise-induced glucose uptake. It is well known that the concentration, number, affinity, and binding capacity of receptor sites are altered by signals emerging from both the intracellular and extracellular environments (Sutton 1983). Such factors contribute to a more intricate and complex regulatory process involving the physiology of glucose uptake by muscle cells.

There are several hormones which appear to play a role during the stress of physical exercise. The hormones secreted by the various endocrine glands that regulate the changes in carbohydrate and fat metabolism during exercise include the pancreatic hormones, insulin and glucagon, the catecholamines, epinephrine and norepinephrine, and to a minor extent, cortisol, growth hormone (Sutton 1983), and perhaps even thyroxine.

Insulin enhances the synthesis of glycogen in both the liver and in muscles. Insulin acts to enhance glucose uptake by muscle, as described earlier, and it also acts to inhibit the release of free fatty acids from adipose tissue. Since, in exercise, the secretion of insulin is either maintained or somewhat depressed, the free fatty levels rise in the circulation (Sutton 1983). Liver and muscle glycogenolysis is also enhanced so that a greater amount of glucose is released into the circulation (Sutton 1983). Therefore, during exercise, both carbohydrate metabolism (glycogenolysis) and fat metabolism (lipolysis) rapidly increase. Also, at the onset of exercise there is a transient but short decrease in blood glucose. This phenomenon contributes to the increase in pancreatic glucagon secretion.

Glucagon acts to activate glycogenolysis in the liver (Kibler et al. 1984). Glucagon is a hormone that mobilizes glucose from the liver and contributes toward increasing the circulating levels of glucose. The extra glucose is of course needed by muscles. However, it is the acceleration in fat metabolism, rather than carbohydrate metabolism, that becomes the chief source of calories in exercise, particularly in light exercise.

The sympathetic nervous system also contributes to a change in metabolism during exercise. Activation of the sympathetic nervous system results in the stimulation of the adrenal medullary hormones, the catecholamines, norepinephrine and epinephrine. These circulating catecholamines stimulate liver glycogenolysis and hepatic glucose release similiar to that of glucagon, contributing to the elevation in blood glucose levels. These hormones also act to enhance adipose tissue lipolysis, contributing to the rapid rise of free fatty acids into the circulation. Finally, epinephrine also plays a role in inhibiting the secretion of insulin by the pancreas.

Subsequent to the initial increase in lipolysis that occurs during exercise, growth hormone levels increase in the circulation, at least within an hour. Growth hormone may act to stimulate the continuation of lipolysis.

TABLE 2.2. Summary of the Autonomic Nervous System and Endocrine System Response to Exercise

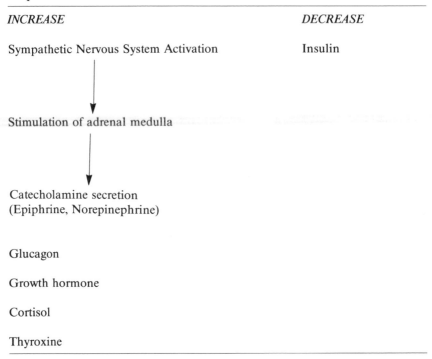

INCREASE	*DECREASE*
Sympathetic Nervous System Activation	Insulin
Stimulation of adrenal medulla	
Catecholamine secretion (Epiphrine, Norepinephrine)	
Glucagon	
Growth hormone	
Cortisol	
Thyroxine	

The adrenal cortex increases its secretion of cortisol during exercise. Cortisol appears to act synergistically with epinephrine in potentiating glycogenolysis in the liver.

Growth hormone and cortisol may also act in concert to depress the secretion of insulin. It appears that both hormones affect insulin receptor activity. Growth hormone decreases the concentration of receptor and cortisol decreases receptor affinity (Sutton 1983).

Another hormone, thyroxine, may also play a role in exercise. A rise in the levels of free fatty acids, such as occurs during exercise, elevates the levels of circulating thyroxine. The elevated levels of thyroxine increase the sensitivity of adipose tissue to the influence of the catecholamines, and therefore enhance catecholamine-induced lipolysis. After exercise ceases, lipolysis continues while fat utilization stops. Therefore, free fatty acids may continue to increase in the circulation at least for a brief period of time following exercise.

There are other hormonal and metabolic changes to consider. With less intense exercise, circulating insulin and glucose levels gradually decline (Sutton 1978). This is accompanied by increasing levels of

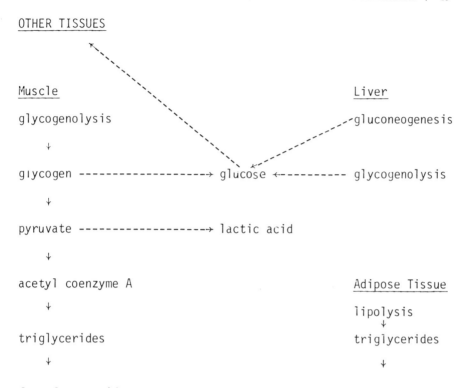

Figure 2.1. Intracellular and extracellular sources of fuel and energy during exercise.

pancreatic glucagon secretion (triggered by a fall in plasma glucose). Glucagon increases blood glucose via glycogenolysis in the liver, as described earlier. The fall in plasma insulin would release the insulin mediated inhibition of adipose tissue lipolysis, thereby enhancing fatty acid metabolism and free fatty acid release into the circulation. Also, in less intense exercise, the change in catecholamine secretion may not be very marked (Sutton 1983).

During intense physical exercise, there is a greater production of lactic acid by muscle cells. The release of lactic acid into the circulation may exert a greater inhibitory effect on adipose tissue lipolysis than the circulating levels of insulin. Also, during intense exercise there is a significant elevation in norepinephrine and epinephrine (Galbo et al. 1975). Blood sugar levels are greatly elevated. This is a result of a more rapid rate of glycogenolysis, which releases glucose into the blood stream, as compared to cellular glucose uptake. Growth hormone and cortisol are secreted in greater amounts during more intense physical exercise.

Therefore, the presence and concentration of the various hormones mentioned depends on the intensity of exercise (Sutton 1983).

A summary of the autonomic nervous system changes and hormonal changes that occur as a result of exercise are shown in Table 2.2. The changes which occur in the metabolic fuels as a result of exercise are shown in Figure 2.1.

SUMMARY

There are several interacting control factors involved in the many changes that take place in the various systems of the body during the stress of physical exercise in normal subjects, many of which are not completely understood (Roth and Grunfeld 1981). Numerous enzymatic reactions taking place in proper sequence, and the central nervous system coordinated control of all the major systems in the body is involved. Studies in the literature report slight variations in the secretions of the various hormones during physical exercise as a function of the physical state of the subject, which includes such factors as habitual exercise, trained vs. untrained, and normal weight vs. overweight or obesity (Richard et al. 1982). All of these factors can result in slight changes in the hormones secreted during exercise as compared to a control population. As discussed in the text, other types of stress, such as trauma and emotional reactivity, as well as physical exercise will stimulate the activity of the central nervous system, sympathetic nervous system, and the adrenal medulla. The general outcome is the enhanced secretion of catecholamines. It is interesting to note that growth hormone, cortisol, and glucagon have also been shown to be increased not only during the stress of physical exercise but also during several other types of stress exposure. The reactions of the physical body to these various types of stress appear to be very much the same as during physical exercise, with one exception—there is no initial rapid utilization of free fatty acids and glucose.

Exercise, whether acute or prolonged, light or strenuous, involves changes in metabolism, body temperature, respiration, circulation, and the cardiovascular system. In addition, sequential enzymatic reactions, hormonal changes, and nervous system (central and autonomic) regulation all contribute and interact in a precise, dynamic way to allow for the physiological adjustments necessary in exercise.

It goes without saying that a regular program of physical exercise can help build a healthy body. Exercise, besides enhancing the tone and quality of the muscular system, adds to the strength, vitality, and integrity of the other organ systems of the body as well. Exercise stimulates blood flow, enhancing oxygen transfer to the various tissues and organs of the body. Stimulation of the lymph system also occurs. Metabolism, digestion, and elimination are stimulated and the lungs and heart are strengthened. Several studies in humans and animals report that exercise can be protective against heart disease caused by the clogging of coronary arteries by cholesterol. Exercise appears to dilate coronary arteries and therefore increases coronary blood flow. Exercise aids in the development of body symmetry as well as enhancing body coordination, balance, and poise. Exercise stimulates the mind and the emotions in positive and healthful directions.

There are various types of physical exercises that one can engage in. It is beyond the scope of this book to enter into a detailed description of any of these exercises, but a chosen exercise program should fit the needs of the individual. Any exercise program when first initiated should be light and gradually increased in heaviness. Exercise should be performed either before meals or at least an hour after meals so as not to hamper the process of digestion. Physical exercise should be engaged in regularly along with a balanced diet of nutritionally healthy foods.

3

VITAMINS

INTRODUCTION

Vitamins belong to a group of organic substances that form an integral and necessary part of the various chemical reactions involved in normal metabolism. Vitamins are absolutely essential for the normal functioning of a healthy body. These substances are present in minute amounts such as milligrams (thousandths of a gram) or even, in some cases, units of micrograms (millionths of a gram). Although the body itself is composed of less than one percent vitamins, the absence of these vitamins or micronutrients in the diet leads to the onset of various deficiency diseases.

The human body is not equipped with the machinery to synthesize most of the vitamins, so they must be obtained from external food sources, both plant and animal. The different vitamins are found in different food groups. While several types of foods supply various types and amounts of vitamins, no one type of food supplies all of the vitamins.

Vitamins cannot be considered sources of energy. They do not have any caloric value. They act mainly in a capacity as regulators of those chemical reactions involved in metabolism, and therefore they are absolutely indispensable for the maintenance of health. In their role as regulators, they are involved in energy transformations, often acting as coenzymes in various enzymatic reactions. They generally act as catalysts in almost all the various chemical reactions involved in metabolism. While catalysts do not participate in chemical reactions, their presence is absolutely necessary for chemical reactions to occur.

The chemical nature and structure of most of the vitamins are known. Most of them have been isolated and some of them have been synthesized. They all differ from each other in chemical composition and in the types of metabolic reactions in which they participate in the body. All of the vitamins are unstable and can easily be destroyed in the presence of such factors as oxygen (when it leads to oxidation), light, heat, and strong acids. Some of the vitamins are soluble in water and some of them are soluble in fat. Stress may influence the activity of vitamins. Other conditions may prevail in which some vitamins fail to be absorbed in the body. For example, if for some reason the digestion of fat is impaired, the fat-soluble vitamins may not be able to be reabsorbed and therefore be used by the body.

Many of the vitamins differ from one another in chemical composition. However, some of them, such as vitamins A, D, E, and K, consist of several closely related compounds that behave similarly and exert similar physiological effects. Also, the B complex vitamins are grouped together, not so much because they consist of a group of closely related compounds but because they generally are found together in specific food groups.

The vitamins not only play a very important role in the regulation of specific metabolic processes in the body but they also play an important role in the prevention of disease. The lack of certain amounts of vitamins in the body result in the onset of various deficiency diseases. A specific deficiency disease is caused by a lack of a specific vitamin. The deficiency diseases associated with the lack of each specific vitamin will be briefly discussed in the sections that follow.

Although the human body does not generally manufacture the necessary amounts of vitamins that it needs, vitamins A, D, K, and nicotinic acid can be manufactured in the body from precursor substances or provitamins. For example, the carotenes found in the body undergo conversion to vitamin A. The interaction of ultraviolet light on the skin can result in the formation of vitamin D. The amino acid tryptophan can be converted to nicotinic acid, which is part of the B complex vitamins. The symbiotic relationship of bacteria in the intestine can result in the formation of vitamin K. The bacterial flora in the gastrointestinal tract are also capable of manufacturing such vitamins as nicotinic acid, folic acid, riboflavin, and vitamin B_{12}. Since the large intestine contains most of the bacterial flora, and since absorption in the large intestine is specifically characterized by electrolyte and water reabsorption, the presence of such bacteria may play a minor role in the amounts of certain vitamins available in the body. However, when an intestinal disorder is present, which may occur as a result of a nutritional or a stress-related condition, an unusually large amount of bacteria may be present in the intestinal tract that are not normally present in the healthy state. The presence of such bacteria may affect the availability of vitamins in the body by decreasing their amounts rather than increasing them. Hence a nutritional disorder or stress, whether acute or chronic, if it results in an increase in parasympathetic activity to the extent of producing diarrhea, may in the short or long term result in a decrease in the availability of certain vitamins in the body.

While all the vitamins perform specific functions, they do not function entirely individually. They are often interrelated in their reactions with other vitamins or other nutrients. For example, excessive amounts of vitamin C and vitamin E may interfere with the body's use of vitamin A. Vitamin E usually functions in conjunction with the trace mineral selenium. This is very similar to the situation that exists between the different hormones in the body. While each hormone produces a specific physiological effect, no hormone really acts alone. Each hormone produces its effect in the presence of other, permissive, hormones.

A summary depicting both the sources and U.S. recommended daily allowances for the various vitamins is presented in Table A-I of the Appendix.

FAT-SOLUBLE VITAMINS

Four known fat-soluble vitamins are considered essential to human health. Three of these, vitamins A, D, and E, must be obtained from external food sources and can be found listed in the "Recommended Dietary Allowances of the National Research Council" (1980). Vitamin K, the fourth vitamin, is also vital to human health but it is synthesized in the body.

Since these four vitamins are fat-soluble, they share some characteristics. For example, they are somewhat stable in the presence of heat. The vitamin content of foods containing these vitamins will be little affected by ordinary cooking temperatures or food processing.

The fat-soluble vitamins are absorbed in the gastrointestinal tract along with fats. Any condition that would limit or compromise fat absorption will also influence the absorption of the fat-soluble vitamins.

VITAMIN A

Introduction

Vitamin A or retinol (A_1) is not synthesized in the human body and therefore must be obtained from food sources of animal origin or from supplements. Mammals and salt-water fish are the main source of vitamin A. The livers of fresh-water fish also contain a form of vitamin A referred to as vitamin A_2. Vitamin A_2 has similar properties to vitamin A_1, but has only about half the biological activity.

While retinol is found only in the animals just mentioned, vitamin A precursors (provitamins), such as the carotenes and carotenoids, are found only in plants. These precursors serve as the primary source of vitamin A for animals. They are found mainly in green and yellow plants and form the yellow pigments of most vegetables and fruits. The conversion of these precursor substances to vitamin A in the animal probably takes place in the intestine.

In the human body, vitamin A and the carotenes, when present in amounts in excess of body needs, are stored in the liver.

Physiological Functions

The importance of this vitamin to human health cannot be overestimated. It appears to be necessary for normal growth, normal bone development, the formation of teeth, healthy skin, the repair of body tissue, and the proper development of epithelial cells. Epithelial cells serve an important function since they line the respiratory and urinary tracts, form the outer layer of the skin, and in some organs and tissues of the body are specialized for transport and secretion. Vitamin A is essential for maintaining the integrity of the mucous membranes that line the mouth, nose, throat, lungs, ears, and other body organs. Vitamin A is required for normal vision and for maintaining good vision, particularly in dim light. It also appears to play a role in reproduction.

Deficiency Disorders

Hypovitaminosis A, or a lack of vitamin A in the body, interferes with the process of growth. There is also a decrease in the resistance of the body to infections. This may occur as a result of the role that vitamin A plays in maintaining the integrity of the epithelial cells. Epithelial cells in the body that specialize in the secretion of mucus may be impaired in their function when vitamin A is not present in sufficient amounts. The mucous membranes serve as a protective barrier against several types of invasive bacteria. As a result, a lack of vitamin A may result in respiratory infections and infections of the nasal and ear cavities.

A deficiency in vitamin A may also cause the various epithelial cells of the body to lose their normal soft and moist status and become somewhat hard and dry. This situation can easily result in a decrease in mucus and other necessary formation and secretion of body fluids. This condition is known as keratinization. The skin may therefore become rugged and dry and blemished as a result of vitamin A deficiency.

Calcium metabolism, and therefore the development of bone, cartilage, and teeth, may be impaired by a lack of vitamin A. Vitamin A plays a role, along with vitamin C and D, in the formation of bones and teeth.

Lack of vitamin A may interfere with the intestinal flora and result in damage to the gastrointestinal tract. Vitamin A works in association with vitamin B to maintain the integrity of the digestive system.

A severe form of vitamin A deficiency is known as xerophthalmia. It is associated with a defect of the eye and with malnutrition. This condition is not very common in the United States and other western countries, but is found more in several of the countries of Asia and the Middle East. A mild deficiency of vitamin A in humans can cause night blindness, conjunctivitis, and possible keratinization of the cornea. Xerosis is a condition in which the eyeball becomes dry and inflamed and loses its characteristic luster, and vision is somewhat impaired. A more severe deficiency can result in keratomalacia (a softening of the cornea) and permanent blindness.

Toxicity

Excess amounts of vitamin A is referred to as hypervitaminosis A. It can occur when an acute dose is ingested, which is extremely high relative to body weight, or when a chronic dose in excessive amounts is ingested over a prolonged period.

The symptoms include drowsiness, nausea, vomiting, headache, and gastrointestinal disturbances, including diarrhea. In chronic cases, other symptoms become manifest, such as irritability, anorexia, dry itching skin, skin rashes, coarse hair, hair loss, blurred vision, swellings at the extremities and over the long bones, and growth depression.

Vitamin A and Stress

Several researchers have studied the effects of acute and chronic stress on the changes that occur in the blood levels, tissue levels, and excretion of vitamin A, in both animals and humans. Some of the stressors studied include emotional stress (Hepner and Maiden 1971), physical training (Barisov 1977), surgery and myocardial infarction (Ramsden et al. 1978), and heat and cold stress (Porter and Masoro 1961; Page et al. 1959; Sundaresan et al. 1967). Several of these researchers found the serum concentrations of vitamin A to fall in both animal and human subjects exposed to these types of stressors.

The effects of other types of stress on vitamin A levels in the body have also been studied. Studies in laboratory animals indicate a direct relationship between vitamin A and protein metabolism. For example,

Deshmukh et al. (1964) subjected rats to the nutritional stress of protein deficiency and found that vitamin A absorption was depressed. Also, plasma vitamin A concentrations were found to be quite low in kwashiorkor infants (Arroyane et al. 1961; Reddy and Srikantia 1966; Reddy 1981). Rechcegl et al. (1962) showed that liver storage, use, and mobilization of vitamin A was reduced under conditions of low dietary protein intake. Surekha et al. (1974) demonstrated that rats fed a deficient protein diet had a greater content of vitamin A per gram of tissue in both the liver and the kidney than did control rats. However, the vitamin A content of the total liver decreased. This appears to be related to the fact that during different stages of protein deficiency, the increase of vitamin A is much smaller over time. Also, the plasma contained less vitamin A than in the control rats. These studies indicate that the liver's use of vitamin A as well as absorption is markedly decreased in protein-deficient rats. In their repletion studies, these researchers found that vitamin A levels of all three tissues became comparable to those of normal rats. Their experiments clearly demonstrate that the steps regulating vitamin A metabolism in animals are influenced by the nutritional stress of protein malnutrition. These researchers indicate that it is conceivable that a similar situation occurs in protein deficiency in humans and that repletion can reverse the ill effects of protein deficiency. Their studies stress the importance of feeding kwashiorkor infants with vitamin A deficiency a high-protein diet along with vitamin A supplementation.

Nakano and Morita (1982) studied the redistribution of vitamin A in tissues of rats exposed to chronic confinement stress. These researchers demonstrated that chronic stress causes a lowering of the serum content of vitamin A. They also found an accumulation of vitamin A in the adrenal gland during immobilization stress, even through the laboratory animals were fed a vitamin A–free diet. Their results are in agreement with others (Glick et al. 1966), who also observed increases in adrenal vitamin A in animals undergoing the stress of foot-shock combined with fasting. Sundaresan and Sundaresan (1975) found a rapid accumulation of vitamin A in the adrenal glands of vitamin A–deficient rats when given a small amount of the vitamin. In accord with these results, all these researchers suggest a significant involvement of vitamin A in the adrenal gland. Perhaps this vitamin is directly implicated in the regulation of steriod hormone synthesis and release. It has also been observed that a deficiency of vitamin A leads to a rapid loss of vitamin C.

Nakano and Morita (1982) studied the content of vitamin A, as a result of chronic immobilization stress, in other tissues. They found large changes in the vitamin A content of kidneys and no significant change of vitamin A content in liver and testes. Nakano and Morita report that feeding rats a vitamin A–free diet results in a distinct elevation of the vitamin A content of the kidneys. The imposition of stress on these same rats, however, greatly inhibited the increase in the vitamin A content of the kidneys. In another study, Ramsden et al. (1978) found that men experiencing the stress of surgery exhibit a decline in their serum content of vitamin A. These researchers suggest this may be the result of an incidental urinary loss of the vitamin. They suggest that the stress-induced decrease in the content of vitamin A in the kidneys may not primarily be a result of a decrease in the serum content of the vitamin, but rather may be a result of an increase in urinary loss. It is the increase in urinary loss that causes the observed lowering of serum vitamin A content of the kidneys.

Morita and Nakano (1982), in another study, report the influence of consecutive daily immobilization stress on vitamin A distribution in tissues of rats fed an adequate vitamin A diet. Their results show that chronic immobilization stress influences vitamin A content of the serum, kidneys, liver, testes, and adrenal glands. In this study, they report significant reductions in vitamin A concentrations of serum, kidneys, and total vitamin A content of the testes. There was a slight reduction in liver vitamin A content. On the other hand, the amount of vitamin A content of the adrenal glands increased. This finding is in agreement with their previous work. These researchers propose that the changes in adrenal vitamin A content may be a reflection of the enlargment of the organ as a result of stress. They also state that the changes that occur in vitamin A content of the kidney, testes, and adrenal glands are most likely produced by the stress itself, rather than by any possible decrease in dietary vitamin A intake, which may be reflected by a decrease in liver vitamin A content. These researchers conclude that a reduction in blood vitamin A as a result of chronic immobilization stress may have been caused by an increase in either urinary loss or by its removal by the adrenal glands. They indicate that these results most likely reflect the changes in the metabolism of vitamin A of these tissues. Morita and Nakano found serum vitamin A levels to fall from a control level of 60 g/dl to 30 g/dl, which, they state, can be regarded as a manifestation of the stress response. As a result of their work these researchers contend that blood vitamin A levels could serve as a useful diagnostic measure to assess the state of the stress response in both human and animals.

Another study concerned with vitamin A and stress discusses the factors involved in the pathogenesis of atherosclerosis. Atherosclerosis is a disease characterized by damage or lesions of the arterial walls. This occurs as a result of an accumulation of a number of substances along the arterial walls, including fibrous tissue, calcium, blood products, and, most particularly, lipid and cholesterol deposits. This abnormal accumulation of substances is probably one of the most important factors in the genesis of the disease. Vitamin A supplementation has been shown to enhance serum lipids in some animal species. On the other hand, Wood and Topliff (1961) show that vitamin A supplementation decreases serum cholesterol levels. Kinley and Krause (1959) also show that vitamin A supplementation can reduce hypercholesterolemia in humans.

In view of this research, Krause et al. (1968) studied the effect on the lipid content of various tissues through the administration of dietary factors that induce atherogenic stress and subsequent vitamin A supplementation. These researchers applied ACTH (adrenocorticotropic hormone), thiouracil, and a high fat diet (all atherogenic factors) to purebred beagle dogs. As a result, the lipid characteristics of the serum and tissues changed in the following ways: (1) total serum lipids increased; (2) all organ triglycerides increased and organ phosopholipids decreased; (3) amounts of saturated fatty acids associated with esterified lipids were increased; and (4) free cholesterol associated with arterial segments increased. These researchers found that subsequent vitamin A supplementation altered the changes in lipid content of various tissues brought on by atherogenic stress. Vitamin A was shown to (1) elevate all serum lipids above atherogenic levels with one exception, that of cholesterol, (2) increase all organ content of phospholipid, and (3) reduce percentages of saturated fatty acids in esterified lipid, and (4) increase all arterial lipid levels except that of free cholesterol, which was lowered. As a result of this work, Krause et al. (1968) conclude that vitamin A tends to enhance lipid storage in all tissues studied except arteries. In arterial segments, the only apparent usefulness of vitamin A during atherogenic stress is to slow down the deposit of free cholesterol.

Vitamin A has been shown to exert a positive effect against experimental gastric stress ulcer (Martin et al. 1967; Moacelli and Pala 1969) and excessive burn injury (Chernov et al. 1969, 1971). These researchers report that in a control group, stress ulcers occurred in 63 percent of the cases, while in those patients who were under vitamin A supplementation only 18 percent exhibited the malady.

Kasper et al. (1975) investigated the concentration of serum vitamin A and its carrier proteins, retinol-binding protein and prealbumin, in response to stress in humans. They found that the serum concentration of vitamin A and both its carrier proteins was significantly decreased after trauma and surgery. These researchers also evaluated the relationship between gastrointestinal hemorrhage and the concentrations of vitamin A in the serum. Gastrointestinal hemorrhages were associated with either extremely low serum vitamin A concentrations or with values lying in the lower normal range. While it is known that vitamin A is necessary for the normal functioning and replication of mucus-secreting epithelia, the mechanism underlying the protective nature of vitamin A in reducing the development of stress-induced gastric ulcers in both laboratory animals and humans remains to be clarified.

Vitamin A has also been implicated in playing a role in other types of stress exposure, particularly, those associated with states of immuno-suppression. Several studies describe the effects of various types of chronic stress exposure on laboratory animals. In some cases thy-molymphatic atrophy (a shrinkage of the thymus gland) and adrenal cortical hypertrophy (enlargement of the adrenal cortex) occur. A detailed description of this phenomenon is given in the pioneering classical experiments of Selye (1956) and also in the work of Santisteban (1953), Dougherty and White (1945), and recently Riley (1975). In such cases, an immunosuppression occurs that appears to be mediated through increased adrenal corticosterone production, with subsequent increased levels of the hormone in the blood stream. The animals develop an immunosuppression or weakened immune system (a reduced state of immunocompetence) and become more susceptible to noxious agents.

Several articles exist which describe the effects of stress exposure on tumorgenesis and cancer development in laboratory animals (Riley 1975). Studies described by Seifter (1976); and Seifter et al. (1973a, 1973b, 1973c) demonstrate such physiological changes in mice exposed to oncogenic viruses. Seifter et al. (1973b) and Zisblatt et al. (1973) found that vitamin A blocks some of the host responses to the stress exposure of tumor-producing viruses. In particular, vitamin A was found to be protective to the host against both thymic involution and tumor development. Rettura et al. (1975) demonstrate that vitamin A alone, without the presence of any other chemotherapeutic agent, inhibits the growth of transplanted tumor cells. Felix et al. (1975) also report a decrease in tumor incidence in virus-injected mice treated with vitamin A compared to untreated mice that eventually died of melanoma.

Along the same vein, other researchers have studied the effects of vitamin A and its possible role in decreasing the incidence of cancer. Sporn et al. (1976) and McCormick et al. (1981) studied the effects of vitamin A supplementation on chemical-, virus-, and radiation-induced cancers in laboratory animals. These researchers found the incidence of cancer to be reduced upon treatment with vitamin A. Also, Wald et al. (1980) and Kark et al. (1981) report two epidemiological studies in which human subjects were treated with high serum vitamin A levels with subsequent reduced risk of cancer. However, Willett et al. (1984), in their study with human subjects, failed to confirm previous reported ob-servations that low levels of vitamin A are related to the incidence of cancer. Their conclusions are the same for vitamin E as well. They do contend however, that their experimental results do not rule out the possibility that these nutrients may have a protective influence on certain subgroups of the population or against particular types of cancers.

These and other similar studies point to the necessity of investigating the potential use of vitamin A as a protective measure against the dangerous and lethal effects of stress. The therapeutic implications should be considered important and worthy of further investigation.

The literature provided by the Committee on Diet, Nutrition and Cancer (1982) demonstrates that indeed there is a large and continually growing body of evidence to suggest that not only vitamin A but various other dietary factors may have an impact on human cancer.

In summary, many types of stress exposure have been shown to lower blood vitamin A levels. Vitamin A is shown to act as a stimulant for both the adrenal and thyroid glands, both of which play important roles maintaining metabolism. Also, activation of these glands stimulates vitamin A production. During cold stress, the body's need for vitamin A is increased. Vitamin A stimulates the activity of the thyroid and adrenal glands, thereby increasing metabolism and body heat. The presence of vitamin A is also necessary for the synthesis of the stress hormones of the adrenal gland. These adrenal hormones aid the body in gearing up for emergency conditions in states of stress. Therefore, in conditions of stress, especially chronic stress, vitamin A supplementation is recommended, since it is being used by the body rapidly and in greater amounts.

VITAMIN D

Introduction

Vitamin D is another vitamin that is soluble in fat and insoluble in water. It has been shown to be strongly associated with the minerals calcium and phosphorus. Hence it is a vitamin necessary for the development of good bone structure.

The vitamin D complex consists of several substances, but as far as human nutrition and therapeutics are concerned, two forms—vitamin D_2 (a synthetic) and vitamin D_3 (formed in the body)—are the most important. Vitamin D_2 is produced by exposing a sterol, called ergosterol, which is found in both yeast and fungi, to irradiation by ultraviolet light. Several substances are produced by such a process, many of which are toxic. However, an important byproduct, ergocalciferol, or vitamin D_2, is produced and has applications in human therapeutics. It is particularly used in the prevention of rickets and is therefore known for its antirachitic effects.

Vitamin D_3, or cholecalciferol, is also produced on exposure to ultraviolet light. This vitamin is manufactured from a sterol, known as 7-

dehydrocholesterol, a derivative of cholesterol, which is widely found in animal fats. A good example is its presence in the oily secretions of mammalian skin.

Ultraviolet rays are important in Vitamin D production; they are found in sunlight. The intensity of these rays varies from the tropic to the temperate zones, being of course more intense in the tropics than in temperate climates. Altitude is also an important consideration. There is a greater exposure to these rays in mountainous regions than at lower outlying plains, valleys, or even at sea level. Clothing, dust, glass windows, and weather conditions (clouds, fog, etc.) absorb ultraviolet rays. Therefore, it is important to take all these factors into consideration when considering surroundings that would be favorable for sunlight to activate the production of vitamin D_3 in the body.

Vitamin D_2 occurs only rarely in nature. It is present in small amounts in certain liver oils of fish but is absent in almost all plant and animal tissues. As previously stated, ergosterol, the substance from which it is manufactured, is found only in plants, that is, yeasts and fungi.

Vitamin D_3, on the other hand, is widely distributed in certain animals fats. In humans, vitamin D_3 is mainly formed by the action of ultraviolet light on the skin. This is the way most human beings satisfy their requirements for vitamin D. Both human and cow's milk contain negligible amounts of this vitamin.

Physiological Functions

Vitamin D is vital for maintaining the proper ratio of calcium and phosphorous in the body. It is therefore necessary not only for the formation of bone but for the healthy development and mineralization of the skeleton and teeth, and thus is crucial to the health of growing children. Vitamin D has as its main site of action the small intestine, where it enhances the absorption of calcium and phosphorous from the gut. It exerts a direct influence on bones, the kidneys, and perhaps several other tissues in the body, appearing to work in conjunction with parathyroid hormone in the regulation of the blood levels of calcium and phosphorous. Vitamin D helps to promote the urinary tubular absorption of phosphate. In humans, one of the early events in the development of rickets is an increase in the urinary levels of phosphate and a decrease in the phosphate plasma levels. These two events could very well disturb the mineralization of bone. Vitamin D is necessary for the prevention of rickets in infants and children and osteomalacin in adults.

Deficiency Disorders

The main vitamin D deficiency disease is rickets. This disease occurs mainly in children and is caused by a lack of absorption of calcium and phosphorus from the intestine and the reabsorption of phosphate by the renal tubules. As a result, a deficient deposit of calcium and phosphates can occur in developing bone and cartilage. Abnormalities in bone structure and severe tooth decay could be the outcome.

Osteomalacia occurs in adults and is characterized by a softening of the bones. Women living in certain parts of the world who have had many pregnancies and who live on a meager diet are particularly prone to this disease. It is not a serious problem in the United States due to the presence of adequate amounts of sunlight and fortified milk.

Toxicity

Caution should be taken when ingesting extra doses of vitamin D. The fat-soluble vitamins take a longer time to be metabolized in the body and then eliminated as compared to the water-soluble vitamins. Excessive vitamin D accumulating in the body may result in toxic side effects, such as abnormal calcium deposits in the walls of blood vessels, lungs and kidneys. Unusual thirst, itching of the skin, and gastrointestial distress symptoms such as loss of appetite, nausea and vomiting, abdominal cramps, weakness, fatigue, irritability, and dizziness may occur.

Vitamin D and Stress

Vitamin D is necessary for maintaining a stable nervous system, normal heart function, and normal functioning of the blood-clotting mechanism. All of these physiological states are associated with the supply and use of calcium and phosphorus by the body. Vitamin D therefore plays an important role in the body's metabolism of calcium.

There is little research available which indicates any direct relationship between levels of vitamin D in the body and various types of stress exposure. Perhaps any relationship between vitamin D and stress may involve the more direct effects of stress on calcium and phosphorus levels in the blood. In view of this, vitamin D would be of benefit in times of stress. Vitamin D has been used along with vitamin A in the treatment of some forms of chronic asthma, arthritis, and chronic anxiety depression (Reich 1975).

VITAMIN E

Introduction

Evans and Bishop (1923), through their experimentation on laboratory rats, discovered a substance with sterility properties. They fed both male and female rats a specific purified laboratory diet and found that these animals failed to reproduce even though they continued to grow. Their diet consisted of lard, butter, cornstarch, and other foods. The sterility condition was corrected when a diet consisting of yeast, fresh lettuce, wheat, oats, and other food supplements were fed to the rats. These experiments were a prelude to the discovery of vitamin E. In 1924, vitamin E was given its name. But it was not until 1936 that the tocopherols (vitamin E) were isolated in pure form from wheat germ oil concentrates.

Today, there are at least eight different compounds identified as tocopherols and tocotrienols that have vitamin E activity. While all of these substances have the same physiological properties, *alpha*-tocopherol is by far the most biologically active and most potent. It is this form of the vitamin that is synthesized commercially.

Vitamin E is a fat-soluble compound and is therefore insoluble in water. It is found in all cell membranes of both animals and plants. It is very heat stable even at temperatures above 100°C. It is also stable in the presence of visible light but unstable in the presence of ultraviolet light. All of the tocopherols are noted for their antioxidant properties; that is, they oppose the oxidation of substances whether within the body or outside of it.

Physiological Functions

Vitamin E is found in all tissues of the body but stored mainly in adipose and muscle tissue, the brain, and the adrenal, reproductive, and pituitary glands. As mentioned previously, it is fat-soluble and found in all cell membranes. It therefore appears to play a role in maintaining the integrity of the cell membrane structure.

Vitamin E is an active antioxidant. It essentially prevents the destructive nonenzymatic oxidation of fat compounds, particularly unsaturated fatty acids. Here, the activity of vitamin E is very similar to some products used in the food industry to prevent fats from getting rancid. Vitamin E also prevents the oxidation of other compounds, such as vitamin A, some vitamin C, and selenium. Being an antioxidant, it also aids the red blood cells in maintaining their normal resistance to destruction by various oxidizing agents.

Vitamin E is also a vasodilator and an anticoagulant. Its presence appears to enhance the activity of vitamin A.

While vitamin E has been recommended in the treatment of several functional disorders, it is not clear whether it performs a necessary and vital role in the alleviation of such disorders. Such disorders include amenorrhea, habitual abortion, muscular dystrophies, lack of fertility, skin disorders, the improvement of reproductive performance, and the retardation of the aging process. Several researchers report possible therapeutic roles for vitamin E in the treatment of some myopathies, encephalopathies, certain hereditary deficiencies, cardiovascular diseases, red blood cell abnormalities, and responses to toxic agents (Horwitt 1980).

Deficiency Disorders

Vitamin E is widely distributed in the various types of available foods, so dietary deficiences of this vitamin are not likely to occur.

In some patients, intestinal absorption of fats and oils, and therefore of vitamin E, may be impaired for any number of reasons. Conditions such as liver cirrhosis or cystic fibrosis can result in such a state. Also, in some cases the red blood cells may become more susceptible to hemolysis. Vitamin E supplementation has been observed to improve absorption and to prolong the life of red blood cells.

Vitamin E deficiency may result in anemia and liver and kidney damage. A deficiency of this vitamin may also result in muscle-wasting diseases and reproductive disorders. This vitamin plays an essential role in normal reproduction in many animals. In males, deficiency of vitamin E will result in a general decrease in sexual instincts and nonmotile sperm. In females a deficiency of vitamin E will result in abortion of the fetus approximately at the midterm of pregnancy. In human reproduction, the exact role of this vitamin is at present not precisely clear.

Toxicity

To date, there are no clear indications that vitamin E is toxic even at doses well above the physiological range.

Vitamin E and Stress

Many experiments have verified that vitamin E–deficient animals are more susceptible to the effects of stress exposure than normal animals. Dietary and environmental stresses have been shown to lead to disease and even fatality in vitamin E–deficient animals. Harris and Mason (1956) and Diplock et al. (1967) list several stress factors or stressors that can lead to vitamin E deficiency with its attendant symptoms. Some of the chemical or dietary stressors include vitamin A, sulphonamides, silver salts, alcohol, lead poisoning, and iron toxicity. Some of the environmental stressors include hypoxia (an amount of oxygen below normal levels) and hyperoxia (an amount of oxygen above normal levels). In other words, vitamin E–deficient animals are quite sensitive to a decrease or an increase in oxygen tension (Taylor 1953; Diplock et al. 1967; Jamieson and Van den Brenk 1964).

The stress factor that has been the most widely studied in vitamin E-deficient animals is unsaturated fat in the diet. Many researchers have demonstrated that both unsaturated fat and some specific polyunsaturated fats in the diet lead to a greater deficiency of vitamin E and therefore accelerate vitamin E deficiency diseases in animals (Green and Bunyan 1969). According to Green et al. (1967a), the effects of dietary fat stress in vitamin E-deficient animals may result from a destruction of tocopherol either in the diet or the gastrointestinal tract of the animal and an added requirement for the metabolism of specific long-chain fatty acids by vitamin E.

Along similar lines, Hayes et al. (1969) studied the effect of vitamin E deficiency coupled with fat stress in the dog. These researchers fed dogs a vitamin E-deficient diet that contained a large amount of polyunsaturated fats over a period of time with and without vitamin E supplementation. They reported that the dogs that did not receive vitamin E supplementation developed a vitamin E deficiency that was correlated with red blood cell hemolysis and reduced tocopherol levels in the plasma. These researchers also found evidence of a browning of the intestinal muscularis in the vitamin E-deficient dogs that was related to the dietary intake of polyunsaturated fats. They also found evidence of both neuroaxonal dystrophy and myodegeneration. These researchers conclude that the vitamin E deficiency or the tocopherol requirement was directly related to the consumption of polyunsaturated fats in the diet.

Some researchers have noted changes in the smooth muscle of arteries and pigmentation of small arterial walls in vitamin E-deficient dogs fed a high polyunsaturated fat diet (Cordes and Mosher 1966). Other researchers have investigated the relationship to dietary fats in vitamin E-deficient rats. In particular, Sen (1965) demonstrated a tendency for polyunsaturated fats in the diet to enhance the hemolysis of blood cells. Still other researchers have investigated the occurrence of the brown bowel syndrome in humans (Toffler et al. 1963) and vitamin E deficiency conditions (Bender et al. 1965; Horwitt 1962).

Interrelationships exist between vitamin E and vitamin A. Many scientific studies, starting with work of Moore (1940), have been undertaken to investigate the nature of these interrelationships. While it is now generally agreed that the availability or the storage of vitamin A is enhanced in the presence of vitamin E, the precise interrelationships existing between these two nutrients still remain to be clarified. Green et al. (1967b) summarize such relationships by listing the possible separate effects of vitamin E on the various aspects of vitamin A metabolism.

According to these researchers, such aspects include a vitamin A uptake that by its absorption through the tissues would somehow depend on the presence of vitamin E for its storage in the liver, and a vitamin A use that may be confined to more specific tissues. Also, any possible effects of vitamin E, independent of vitamin A, on tissue metabolism, which may in turn affect vitamin A, should also be considered. Green et al. emphasize that dietary fat intake, vitamin concentration and intake, time intervals involved, as well as interactions in the digestive tract must all be considered in view of the experimental results obtained. For a more detailed description of the work done in this area, see the work of Green et al. (1967b) and Green and Bunyan (1969).

There is also evidence for a dietary relationship and possibly several other interrelationships between the trace element selenium and vitamin E. Evidence exists that selenium has a specific biochemical role that parallels that of *alpha*-tocopherol (Schwartz 1965; Green and Bunyan 1969). For example, it appears that in the chick, vitamin E and selenium potentiate one another (Calvert et al. 1962), while in other animal species they may be additive or synergistic with one another. However, selenium does not function as a substitute antioxidant for vitamin E.

In view of the relationship between selenium and vitamin E, Van Vleet et al. (1977) studied the protective effect of selenium and vitamin E pretreatment against myocardial damage in swine. These reseachers induced cardiomyopathies in swine by administration of cobalt or isoproterenol. They found that swine with inherited stress susceptibility were more likely to develop a greater severity of cardiomyopathy from cobalt or isoproterenol than the swine that were not stress susceptible. The reason for this has not been elucidated. The study of Van Vleet et al. demonstrates that vitamin E and selenium strongly protect the animal from any cobalt-induced cardiomyopathy but offer only slight protection against large doses of isoproterenol. These researchers suggest that the results of this study may eventually have application to humans, particularly in cardiomyopathies that are a result of nutritional deficiencies.

In summary, recent research indicates that when animals are stressed with a diet of polyunsaturated fats, their stores of vitamin E become rapidly depleted. When sufficient amounts of vitamin E are no longer present, its protective antioxidant effect is diminished. What ensues is a series of biochemical reactions that involve the peroxidation of the polyunsaturated fats. This process results in the liberation of free radicals, which may cause cellular and tissue distribution. Blood, nerve, and muscle cells can become so severely damaged that death may ensue.

Anyone exposed to the stress of an excess oxygen environment, such as the astronauts, or anyone exposed to the stress of air pollution containing nitrous oxide toxins and excess oxygen has been shown to benefit from vitamin E supplementation.

There are also substances in the body that are antagonistic to vitamin E and that can cause its depletion. Such substances include thyroid hormones, iron salts, and estrogen. Women using birth control pills have a greater tendency to develop venous blood clots, perhaps because the estrogen in the pill may use vitamin E and therefore deplete its stores from the body.

VITAMIN K

Introduction

Vitamin K was the last fat-soluble vitamin to be discovered (McCollum 1957). It is shown as an antihemorrhagic vitamin since its lack prolongs the clotting time of blood and produces hemorrhages.

Vitamin K is known to exist in two major natural forms, vitamins K_1 and K_2. Vitamin K_1 is the only form of vitamin K that is found in plant food, particularly in leafy vegetables. Vitamin K_2 was originally found in fish meal but was subsequently found to be synthesized by the bacterial flora of the human intestinal tract. Vitamin K_3 also exists, but it is a synthetic manufactured as menadione sodium bisulfite USP. It is used for patients who are unable to synthesize their own vitamin K because they are deficient in an enzyme necessary for the absorption of the fat-soluble vitamins.

The bacteria *Escherichia coli*, which are found in the human large intestine, synthesize the vitamin. This may explain why vitamin K does not appear to be so vital in the diet of human beings.

Physiological Functions

Basically, vitamin K aids blood coagulation. Its presence is necessary for the formation of prothrombin. Prothrombin is a necessary precursor to thrombin formation. Thrombin is an enzyme that reacts with fibrinogen and converts it into fibrin, the substance necessary for the formation of a blood clot. Therefore, a lack of vitamin K would prolong blood-clotting time and could result in hemorrhages.

Vitamin K is also important for normal liver function.

Deficiency Disorders

Infants can develop vitamin K deficiency if not enough intestinal flora are present to synthesize vitamin K. The deficiency can be corrected by vitamin K administration. In adults, since vitamin K is fat-soluble any defect in intestinal absorption of fats may result in vitamin K deficiency. For example, the secretion of bile and bile salts is necessary for the absorption of vitamin K into the system. Any disorder that interferes with bile production or any biliary obstruction would result in a deficiency of vitamin K.

Because of its biological effects, vitamin K would be useful as an anticoagulant agent. It would practically do away with any prolonged bleeding in operations. It is also a therapeutic agent in bleeding diseases, particularly of the newborn.

Toxicity

No known toxic effects are presently associated with vitamin K.

Vitamin K and Stress

A few studies have investigated the effect of stress on alterations in plasma vitamin K levels or on vitamin K–dependent coagulation factors. Vitamin K is necessary for maintaining the integrity of the blood-clotting mechanism.

Cases have been reported in which toxic levels of iron have been found in the blood as a result of a number of causes, the most common being the oral intake of high doses of the element. Iron appears to have a direct effect on the activity of several vitamin K–dependent coagulation factors found in the blood. The stress of acute iron intoxication was studied by some researchers. Wilson et al. (1958) reports a reduction in the activity of a vitamin K–dependent coagulation factor, as well as fibrinogen and prothrombin, in animals given high doses of iron (ferrous sulfate). In humans, a definite hemostatic defect, along with other complications, has been observed in acute iron intoxication (Eriksson et al. 1974; Henriksson et al. 1979). In particular, the research of Evensen et al. (1982) suggests altered functional activity of several vitamin K–dependent coagulation factors as a result of the ingestion of toxic doses of ferrous sulfate. These researchers conclude that the monitoring of vitamin K–dependent coagulation factors may be the most practical method to follow in the management of acute iron intoxication. These studies demonstrate that while the stress of iron toxicity does not directly affect vitamin K itself, it does alter various blood factors dependent on vitamin K activity.

Some researchers have studied the effects of temperature stress on prothrombin time, which is a measure of blood-clotting time. Denyes and Carter (1961) demonstrate prolonged prothrombin times in several animals exposed to the stress of decreased temperatures. Rubenstein and Lack (1960) also demonstrate prolonged increased prothrombin times as a result of the stress of low temperature exposure. An increase in prothrombin time results in a longer time for coagulation to take place and can therefore enhance the possibility of hemorrhage. An increase in hemorrhagic deaths in vitamin K–deficient rats exposed to the stress of elevated temperatures is reported by Mills et al. (1944). Charles and Day (1968) report an increase in prothrombin time in vitamin K–deficient chicks subject to heat stress. They also report that chicks receiving a diet adequate in vitamin K did not experience a corresponding rise in prothrombin or clotting time. The underlying mechanisms involved in the temperature stress–induced changes in clotting time need further clarification; further studies are needed to shed more knowledge on the mechanisms involved.

In summary, any physiological stress, such as a decrease in the secretion of bile salts due to biliary obstruction, can interfere with the absorption of vitamin K and therefore prevent its use by the body. Other stresses, such as industrial air pollution, radiation, and x rays, destroy vitamin K. The excessive use of some drugs, such as the antibiotics, can destroy the normal population of the intestinal flora, thereby interfering with vitamin K use by the body.

4

WATER-SOLUBLE VITAMINS

Water-soluble vitamins, which include the B vitamins and vitamin C, are not stored in the body as are the fat-soluble vitamins. Because excess amounts are eliminated from the body these vitamins must therefore be replaced on a daily basis.

VITAMIN C

Introduction

Vitamin C, or ascorbic acid, is a white crystalline substance that can be considered a carbohydrate since its chemical composition is very similar to that of a simple sugar. This vitamin, while being water-soluble, is very sensitive to oxygen and is easily oxidized. Of all the vitamins, it is the one that can most easily be destroyed. Its potency can diminish in the presence of light and air, and it is destroyed very easily by heat in the presence of oxygen, as in boiling in open cookware. It is stable in dry form and is less affected by heat in an acid solution. As the solution becomes more alkaline, its stability decreases.

In the human body, vitamin C is found in tissues and cells in varying amounts, mainly in the extracellular fluid compartment of the body. The brain, adrenal gland (cortex), pituitary gland, liver, spleen, pancreas, and ovaries also contain large amounts of the vitamin. Any trauma to the body, such as surgery, a burn, or an injury, can lead to a loss of the reduced form of vitamin C from the body. In general, any form of stress results in a rapid and dramatic loss of the vitamin from the body.

Physiological Functions

The primary function of vitamin C is the correction and prevention of scurvy. Scurvy is characterized by an abnormal formation of bones and teeth and hemorrhagic manifestations. The bones become brittle and can easily fracture. This is a result of an interference in collagen formation; collagen is a protein that provides the bones with hardness and elasticity.

Ascorbic acid is necessary for the synthesis and presence of adequate amounts of collagen in connective tissue. Collagen supports tissue structure. Hence adequate amounts of this vitamin are needed for wound healing, since the adequate healing of a wound requires scar formation containing strong connective tissue.

Vitamin C also plays a role as a strong antioxidant. It acts as a reducing agent in the body; that is, it causes oxygen to be removed in various chemical reactions. It protects the integrity of other well-known antioxidants such as vitamins A and E and the essential fatty acids.

In certain instances, vitamin C can act as a coenzyme in specific chemical reactions.

Vitamin C is necessary for normal physiological functioning in the presence of certain disturbances of the gastrointestinal tract, such as the stomach and bowel. It is also necessary as a protective agent in diseases of the liver. It plays a role in body growth, the building of blood, and improvement of appetite. Its presence is necessary in pregnant and nursing women.

Research is not conclusive as to the role that vitamin C plays in several physiological processes of the body, such as in decreasing blood cholesterol levels, preventing several types of viral and bacterial infections, treating, preventing, and curing the common cold, healing wounds and burns, and in lowering the incidence of venous blood clots and impaired adrenal cortical function.

Deficency Disorders

The main deficiency disorders caused by a lack of vitamin C are scurvy, anemia, underdevelopment of bone cells and teeth, injury to blood vessels, prenatal skeletal formation impairment, and under-nutrition. Signs of vitamin C deficiency are tendency to bruising, swollen joints, lowered resistance to infection, and slow healing of wounds. The blood levels of ascorbic acid are also known to be lowered by nicotine.

Toxicity

There are no proven toxic effects of vitamin C. However, excessive or megadoses of the vitamin can cause some unpleasant side effects, such as skin rashes, kidney stones, and diarrhea.

Vitamin C and Stress

Several research reports describe the effects of vitamin C intake during various types of stress exposure in both animals and humans. A sampling of the animal research literature reveals some very interesting information.

Several types of stress exposure are known to result in changes in the ascorbic acid (vitamin C) content of the adrenal glands in laboratory animals. Irwin et al. (1950) exposed animals to temperature stress, and Evans et al. (1967) exposed animals to environmental pollutants. Both studies demonstrate decreased levels of ascorbic acid content of the adrenals. It has been observed that vitamin C is a potent detoxifier. This vitamin appears to negate the destructive effects of several toxic mineral elements, such as lead, mercury, and other industrial pollutants that may prove to be carcinogenic in the long term.

During stress, not only is the adrenal ascorbic acid content decreased, but cholesterol, a precursor of the adrenal cortical hormones, is also depleted. The role of adrenal ascorbic acid in the synthesis of the adrenal cortical hormones is not entirely clear.

To study this problem, Pohujani et al. (1969) investigated the effects of pretreatment with ascorbic acid on adrenal ascorbic acid content and cholesterol content of the rat during stress exposure. These researchers conclude that a possible relationship or linkage exists between ascorbic acid and cholesterol in the adrenal glands.

Kotze (1975) studied the effect of the stress of captivity on vitamin C levels in free-living baboons. This researcher found that under such stressful conditions, serum vitamin C levels decrease and serum cholesterol levels increase. The increase in serum cholesterol may result from a release of cholesterol from the adrenal glands. Kotze further found that an increase in the dietary intake of vitamin C at the beginning of the captivity period decreased the serum cholesterol levels significantly. As a result of further experimentation, Kotze reports a lowering of serum cholesterol levels (hypocholesteremia) by vitamin C only under conditions of stress.

Several researchers have found either increased or decreased levels of serum cholesterol under other physiological conditions. For example, Zaitsev et al. (1964) report a decrease in cholesterol deposits in the aorta after ascorbic acid administration. These researchers found an increase in liver and adrenal cholesterol content with no change in blood cholesterol levels. Spittle (1971), on the other hand, found an increase in serum cholesterol levels after administering 1 gram of vitamin C daily to atherosclerotic patients. This researcher suggests that the serum cholesterol rise may have occurred as a result of the change in the cholesterol deposits in the arterial walls. Willis (1953) found that guinea pigs on an ascorbic acid–deficient diet exhibited the presence of arterial lesions, which would be quickly reversed by administration of ascorbic acid. Several other scientific investigations implicate vitamin C as one of the many factors able to influence the cholesterol levels in serum and in some other tissues. On the other hand, some researchers do not find any effect of vitamin C administration on serum cholesterol levels. For example, Anderson (1975) found no change in serum cholesterol levels upon administering doses of 1 gram per day of vitamin C to 41 patients. Elwood et al. (1970) also did not find a serum hypocholesteremic effect of vitamin C.

Several researchers have found a relationship between various types of stress conditions and changes in the amount of ascorbic acid found in the adrenal glands. In particular, it has been demonstrated that environmental and metabolic stress exposures can result in changes in the ascorbic acid content of the adrenal glands in experimental animals. Changes in environmental temperature, exposure to experimentally produced tobacco smoke, and administration of toxic compounds are stressors that have been shown to have such an effect (Hughes and Nicholas 1971). Hughes and Nicholas studied the effects of caging on adrenal ascorbic acid content of guinea pigs and gerbils. These researchers found that the adrenal gland concentration of ascorbic acid was higher in the individually caged animals than the grouped caged animals. They conclude that the grouped caged animals (crowding) appeared to be more stressed than the individually caged animals. Paré (1964, 1968) also reports increased values of adrenal ascorbic acid in stressed animals as compared to controls and Zakharova (1967) demonstrates a depletion in the level of adrenal ascorbic acid as a result of stress.

Civen et al. (1980) studied the effect of dietary ascorbic acid and vitamin E deficiency on adrenal metabolism and production of corticosterone in laboratory rats. These researchers found that high concentrations of ascorbic acid in the diet blocked the normal stress-induced increase in plasma and adrenal corticosteroid concentration. They confirmed the role that ascorbic acid appears to play in blocking adrenal corticosteroid production in response to stress.

Other researchers have studied the relationship between ascorbic acid and stress ulcer formation. Cheney and Rudrud (1974) report that rats given ascorbic acid in their drinking water before and during periods of food deprivation, had no ulcer formation. On the other hand, Glavin et al. (1978) demonstrate that ascorbic acid failed to provide total protection against stress ulcer formation. Other researchers claim that ascorbic acid is protective against gastric carcinoma (Raineri and Weisburger 1975). Some researchers have claimed that vitamin C offers protection against the common cold (Pauling 1971; Anderson 1975). Other researchers claim that ascorbic acid may have a protective effect against heat stress, while other researchers, including Henschel et al. (1944), do not support such views.

Other conditions of stress have been noted to be associated with increased levels of ascorbic acid in the serum. McGanity et al. (1967) demonstrate that the ascorbic acid blood levels were significantly greater at the end of surgery and dropped below presurgical levels 24 hours after surgery. Ben Nathan et al. (1976) studied the changes in plasma and leucocyte ascorbic acid content in cocks subjected to the stress of short heat exposure. These researchers found an increase in both plasma and leucocyte ascorbic acid content. This was accompanied by an increase in plasma corticosterone and a significant decrease in white blood cell count. The last two changes are good indicators of the stress response.

Another role of ascorbic acid is in the biological inactivation of histamine (Subramanian et al. 1973). Researchers have reported that histamine stimulation and release occurs in several animal species as a result of various types of stress exposure, including cold exposure, toxins, vaccines, and dietary stress (Schayer 1962; Kahlson and Rosengren 1968). Nandi et al. (1974) studied the effect of ascorbic acid on the biological inactivation of histamine under different stress conditions in laboratory animals. These researchers found that the administration of ascorbic acid in large doses during different types of stress exposure results in a significant decrease in urinary histamine levels and therefore an increase in the biological inactivation of histamine. They state that any beneficial effect of large doses of ascorbic acid under different types of stress exposure appears to be due to a biological inactivation of excess histamine produced in response to stress.

The research work discussed so far has concerned itself with the effects of stress on vitamin C in the laboratory animal. Let us review a sampling of the literature describing the use of ascorbic acid in humans when subjected to various types of stress exposure.

Maas et al. (1961) and Hodges (1970) demonstrate that in humans undergoing stress exposure the urinary excretion of ascorbic acid increases.

Mowle (1981) studied the effect of prolonged physical exertion in humans, particularly that associated with long-distance running and a game of Australian Rules football, on vitamin C levels. This researcher found that certain team members had used significant amounts of ascorbic acid as a result of strenuous physical activity. In particular, Mowle reports that one of the athletes who ran a distance of 6.5 kilometers showed a negative balance of ascorbic acid upon examination of the urine, even though, 15 minutes before running, he was given 4 grams of sodium ascorbate orally. This researcher further reports that the same athlete, when maintained on a daily regimen of 6 to 8 grams of ascorbic acid, exhibited increased speed maintenance and endurance. Other researchers working with athletes also found that after the stress of strenuous physical activity ascorbic acid depletion occurred even though gram doses were administered before the onset of strenuous physical activity (Dettman and Zimmerman 1973).

It has been speculated that low circulating levels of ascorbic acid are an indication that an insufficient supply of vitamin C is present in the adrenals to aid in the synthesis of cortisol—a hormone secreted by the adrenal gland as a result of the stress response. Vitamin C is a precursor in the synthesis of cortisol. Cortisol is needed by the body in the initial stages of the stress response in order for the body to adequately buffer itself against the physiological changes that occur as a result of the imposed stress. If adequate amounts of vitamin C are not present, the body would not possess the necessary biochemical machinery for cortisol synthesis and secretion to take place, which would offset the physiological changes that occur as a result of the elicitation of the stress response.

Vitamin C along with vitamin E and the trace element selenium are antioxidants. It has been suggested that the presence of vitamin C in the adrenal gland is necessary to prevent the oxidation of the adrenal medullary catecholamines epinephrine and norepinephrine. The oxidation of these catecholamines would produce a toxic substance in the body with adverse physiological consequences (Lewin 1976). Stone (1976) describes ascorbic acid as exerting a protective effect on circulating levels of catecholamines. This protective effect is diminished as a result of decreased amounts of ascorbic acid in the adrenal gland. Hence it is speculated that this may be one of the precipitating factors in explaining the diminished performance of individuals subjected to the physiological stress of strenuous activity.

There is also speculation that there may be a link between a decrease in plasma vitamin C levels and coronary heart disease in humans.

Plasma vitamin C was found to decrease with age in adults (Brook and Grenshaw 1968) while coronary heart disease increases with age (Goldstein et al. 1973).

Several types of stress exposure are known to decrease the levels of ascorbic acid in the body. Such stressors include infections, some antibiotics, chemicals, various poisons, birth control pills (Dettman 1973), tobacco smoke (Stone 1976; Pellitier 1968), and alcohol (Pauling 1976). Any of these stressors or a combination can result in various levels of depletion of vitamin C (Mowle 1982) and be detrimental to the individual's physiological balance and health. Many researchers believe that vitamin C depletion in both the short and long term can lead to various disease states and perhaps even precipitate a life-crisis situation.

In summary, vitamin C can be labeled a stress vitamin because it is used by the body rapidly under various types of stressful conditions. Since the cellular and tissue requirements for ascorbic acid are increased as a result of increased metabolism, vitamin C appears to be necessary in all types of stress exposure.

Recommended Daily Allowances

The topic of recommended daily allowances for vitamin C has been widely discussed. Linus Pauling (1976) has indicated that the human need for this vitamin should probably be increased, perhaps by a factor of 10 or more. Much investigative work yet needs to be done to come to a clearer understanding of the amount of vitamin C required under normal physiological conditions. Several researchers have found that the vitamin C requirement generally increases under various types of stress. Man-Li S. Yew (1973), working with guinea pigs, found that animals require significantly more ascorbic acid under stressed conditions than under normal conditions. In addition, Yew concludes that for young guinea pigs and similarly for young human beings, the ascorbic acid requirements are much higher than is presently thought. This researcher also states that while individual needs for vitamin C vary over a wide range, it appears that for the young, the need for the vitamin may be as much as 20 times greater than what is presently accepted.

THE B COMPLEX VITAMINS

Introduction

The B complex vitamins consists of 15 or more water-soluble substances that have been isolated from several sources, such as liver, yeast, fungi, molds, and bacteria. The vitamins that belong to the class of B vitamins and that play an important role in humans include:

Vitamin B_1 (thiamine)
Vitamin B_2 (riboflavin, vitamin G)
Vitamin B_5 (pantothenic acid, calcium pantothenate, panthenol)
Vitamin B_6 (Pyridoxine)
Vitamin B_{12} (cyanocobalamin, cobalamin)
Vitamin B_{13} (orotic acid)
Vitamin B_{15} (pangamic acid)
Vitamin B_{17} (laetrile)
Niacin (nicotinic acid, niacinamide, nicotinamide)
Biotin (coenzyme R or vitamin H)
Inositol
para-Aminobenzoic acid (PABA)
Folic acid (folacin)
Choline

These substances are grouped together as the B complex vitamin family because of their close functional relationships. They are found together in the same type of food substances and perform similar functions in the body.

In general, the importance of the B complex vitamins lies mainly in their ability to influence the growth of the organism and to play an important role in the proper functioning of the muscular system, the cardiovascular system, the nervous system, and the endocrine system. They also influence appetite and the functioning of the gastrointestinal system and play a vital role in carbohydrate metabolism and energy production.

Since the B vitamins are water-soluble, they behave like the other water-soluble vitamins in that any excess in the body is excreted and thus the B vitamins must be replenished daily. Each of the B vitamins performs its own specific function in the body, but all the B vitamins are interrelated and interdependent. A deficiency in one specific B vitamin can lead to a deficiency in the other B vitamins.

Many of the B vitamins act synergistically. They are more potent when acting together than when acting alone. Vitamins B_1, B_2, and B_6, for example, when acting together, exert their influence in the body more effectively than when acting separately.

B Complex Vitamins and Stress

Since the B complex vitamins play an important role in maintaining the integrity of the nervous system and metabolism, they are affected by stress.

There is evidence that the levels of the B complex vitamins decrease in the body as a result of the elicitation of the stress response. It is believed that some of the B complex vitamins are involved in the steroidgenesis of cholesterol into cortisol in the adrenal gland. Stress elevates cortisol in the bloodstream. The stress-induced increase in cortisol production may have some bearing on the decrease in available B complex vitamins in the body. Some research describes the effects of stress on some of the B complex vitamins.

Whitehead et al. (1975) describe a study in which chicks were fed eight experimental diets. The research focused on dietary and environmental factors that resulted in an enhanced fatty liver and kidney syndrome. As expected, a high energy, low fat, and low protein diet produced a high level of mortality (18.9 percent). Addition of fat at the expense of carbohydrate reduced mortality from 18.9 to 7 percent. These researchers further report that supplementation of the diet with a mixture of vitamins reduced the mortality to 1 percent, whereas supplementation of the diet with thiamine alone reduced mortality down to 11 percent. The vitamin mixture included vitamins A, D, E, K, and the B vitamins comprising B_{12}, pantothenic acid, nicotinic acid, riboflavin, biotin, folic acid, inositol, and choline.

Several of the B vitamins appear to be involved in the stress of pregnancy. Throughout pregnancy, several of the B vitamins decrease in the serum of the mother and increase in the serum of the infant. At parturition, samples of both mother and infant serum show that B_{12}, B_5, B_1, and folic acid were much higher in the infant than in the mother. The high infant levels and low maternal levels seem to be a result of these vitamins being taken up by the fetus for cellular growth and metabolism (Barker and Frank 1968). A dysfunction of the amino acid tryptophan may occur during pregnancy, which can be overriden by administration of vitamin B_6. Pregnancy may therefore require twice as much or more of an intake of vitamin B_6 by the mother (Barker and Frank 1968).

VITAMIN B_1 (THIAMINE)

The most important role that vitamin B_1 plays in the human body is in carbohydrate metabolism. Thiamine participates in the form of a coenzyme structure that consists of nonprotein organic substances. This coenzyme is essential for the activity of an enzyme system that governs the reactions that bring about the production of carbon dioxide and the release of energy from glucose breakdown or oxidation.

The enzyme known as transketolase necessitates the presence of thiamine as a cofactor. This enzyme can be found in several tissues of the body, including the liver, kidneys, and red blood cells. The presence of this enzyme in the body is essential for the manufacture of certain sugars and, most importantly, for the production of energy. Therefore, thiamine plays an important role in energy production. Transketolase activity can be used diagnostically as a measure to detect thiamine deficiency in the body. Thiamine is also essential for growth and for maintaining the integrity of the digestive, cardiovascular, and nervous systems.

It is not clear whether disorders of the nervous system are due primarily to a deficiency in thiamine or to a combination of thiamine and other factors.

Thiamine has been shown to have a mild diuretic effect.

Oxidation and heat resulting from cooking can easily destroy this vitamin. In the United States, vitamin B_1 is lost mainly through food-processing procedures such as the pasteurization of milk, the canning of meat, and the milling of cereals.

Deficiency Disorders

A deficiency disorder for thiamine or any of the other vitamins may occur either primarily as a result of improper nutrition or secondarily as a result of factors that either increase the demand for the vitamin or interfere with its proper use by the body.

Beriberi is a deficiency disease associated with inadequate nutrition and a lack of vitamin B_1 in the diet. This disease appears to be endemic in the Orient and many islands of the Pacific. It is commonly found in people whose diet has a low protein, low fat, and high carbohydrate content, such as a diet with a large intake of highly milled rice. This kind of diet would require more than normal amounts of thiamine, since it is used as a coenzyme in carbohydrate use. The symptoms of beriberi are cardiovascular changes, edema, and multiple neuritis (inflammation of a nerve or nerves). Stimulants such as caffeine and nicotine, when taken in excess, can result in a thiamine deficiency.

Toxicity

There is no known toxic reaction for this vitamin since any excess is excreted and not stored in any significant degree in the body.

Vitamin B_1 and Stress

There is a greater demand and need by the body for vitamin B_1 during many stressful conditions, including illness, surgery, pregnancy, and lactation. The acute stress of physical exercise can also increase the body's need for vitamin B_1. Exercise requires a great quantity of energy in a short period of time, and vitamin B_1 is important in energy production. This vitamin plays an important role in the function of the nervous system as well as metabolism.

VITAMIN B_2 (RIBOFLAVIN, VITAMIN G)

Vitamin B_2 is an essential ingredient in living cells and is part of a group of enzymes involved in cellular oxidation as a result of the mobilization and use of carbohydrates, fats, and proteins. Therefore, the vitamin is intimately involved in the release of energy by the cell. This vitamin is also essential for growth and for the functioning of a healthy nervous system. Vitamin B_2 may also play a role in reproduction and in the maintenance of healthy skin, hair, and nails, mucous membranes, and good vision.

Deficiency Disorders

There is no definite disease associated with a deficiency of riboflavin in the diet. However, it is possible that a maintained low intake of the vitamin might result in impaired growth or cheilosis. Cheilosis is a condition characterized by a reddened appearance of the lips and fissures at the angles of the mouth. Weakness and lassitude may occur as a result of a riboflavin deficiency.

Toxicity

No toxic effects of riboflavin have been reported.

Vitamin B_2 and Stress

During conditions of stress the body's need for this vitamin is greatly increased. For example, pregnancy and lactation are conditions that require greater amounts of Vitamin B_2. There is a greater need for this vitamin when excess amounts of protein and carbohydrate are consumed. Due to the stress that many people experience as a result of living in our fast-paced society, the most common vitamin deficiency in America today appears to be a vitamin B_2 deficiency.

Unlike thiamine, riboflavin is not destroyed by oxidation, heat (cooking), or acid, but is relatively stable in the presence of these factors. However, it can be destroyed in the presense of an alkali or upon exposure to ultraviolet light (for example, milk in a glass container left in sunlight).

VITAMIN B₅ (PANTOTHENIC ACID, CALCIUM PANTOTHENATE, PANTHENOL)

This vitamin appears to be a constituent of all living organisms. It enjoys a wide distribution in many types of foodstuffs. Hence it is aptly named pantothenic acid, from the Greek for "everywhere." Deficiencies in this vitamin are not too likely to occur unless the diet consists of a high amount of processed foods.

Pantothenic acid is a component of coenzyme A. It functions in the intermediate metabolism of proteins, carbohydrates, and fats, as well as in the synthesis of fatty acids. This vitamin is also involved in many other important chemical reactions in the body.

Vitamin B₅ is a pale yellow oily liquid that has not yet been crystallized. However, the calcium salt of the vitamin does crystallize readily and it is this form that is generally available.

The vitamin is not stable in dry heat, and if temperatures are not varied over a large range little loss of the vitamin occurs upon cooking. It is stable in neutral solutions but is rapidly destroyed in acid or alkaline solutions.

Deficiency Disorders

Since vitamin B₅ is so widely distributed, deficiency disorders in humans have not been definitively described. However, in some animal species disorders have been recorded.

Toxicity

There are no known toxic effects of this vitamin.

Vitamin B₅ and Stress

Vitamin B₅ is considered an important antistress vitamin. During intense stress, the levels of this vitamin in the body have been found to decrease, which results in adrenal exhaustion. Therefore, vitamin B₅ appears to play a role in maintaining the integrity of the adrenal glands. A deficiency of vitamin B₅ appears to be one of the factors involved in the fatigue and exhaustion associated with chronic intense stress. In general, a deficiency of vitamin B_5 results in a decreased tolerance to various types of stress exposures. Along with fatigue, irritability, insomnia, and depression can occur.

Because of the role of vitamin B_5 in intermediate metabolism, the need for it would appear to increase as intermediate metabolism is increased in response to several types of stress exposure.

VITAMIN B_6 (PYRIDOXINE)

Vitamin B_6 itself forms a complex of vitamins in that it consists of three functionally related compounds—pyridoxine, pyridoxal, and pyridoxamine. Pyridoxal and pyridoxamine are the forms of vitamin B_6 normally found in animal foods. Pyridoxine, on the other hand, is normally found in plant food. All three forms of vitamin B_6 are referred to as pyridoxine.

This vitamin was initially identified as a factor that played a role in curing a specific nutritional form of dermatitis in rats.

Investigative efforts concerning vitamin B_6 have shown that it is associated with several enzyme systems in the body. It is involved as a cofactor in chemical reactions that are associated with protein synthesis and nitrogen metabolism. Therefore, when high protein diets are consumed over an extended period of time, the need for this vitamin increases. It is also involved in chemical reactions involving carbohydrate and fat metabolism.

Research indicates that vitamin B_6 plays a role in red blood cell formation: hence a deficiency can lead to anemia. The vitamin also plays a role in the production of antibodies. Other studies show that the vitamin may influence the endocrine system in the production of several important hormones such as the thyroid and adrenal hormones, the gonadotropins, growth hormone, and insulin. Vitamin B_6 is essential for the proper absorption of vitamin B_{12} by the body. It is a natural diuretic and helps in the prevention of water retention. It is also vital in maintaining electrolyte balance. In general, the need for this vitamin appears to increase in times of stress and greater energy production. Vitamin B_6 is fairly stable in the presence of heat and is sensitive to alkaline solution and ultraviolet light.

Deficiency Disorders

Anemia, pigmented dermatitis, weakness, irritability, insomnia, and depression are some of the symptoms that may develop as a result of a deficiency of this vitamin.

Some women taking oral estrogen contraceptives may develop vitamin B_6 deficiency. This may occur because the female sex hormone may activate a liver enzyme system that converts tryptophan, an essential amino acid, into nicotinic acid, which in turn enhances the need for this vitamin. The presence of vitamin B_6 is necessary for this reaction to go to completion.

Sometimes depression in women is alleviated when vitamin B_6 is given. Depression may be associated with the interference of the metabolism of amines in the brain. In particular, the amine involved is 5-hydroxytryptamine, which is a result of the metabolism of tryptophan.

Also, it is possible that approximately 25 percent of the alcoholic population may have a vitamin B_6 deficiency.

Toxicity

No toxic or adverse reactions have been reported upon the administration of pyridoxine to human beings.

Vitamin B_6 and Stress

Insulin, growth hormone, and vitamin B_6 are involved in the regulation of amino acid transport at the cellular level. The stressful state of vitamin B_6 deficiency results in a decrease in the glandular secretion and circulating levels of both growth hormone and insulin (Heindel and Riggs 1978). It has therefore been postulated that vitamin B_6 activity may be mediated through either or both of these hormones. The action of growth hormone on cartilage is mediated through the somatomedins. Kamala et al. (1982) describe the effects of hormonal modifications in the presence of the stress of a vitamin B_6 deficient diet. In particular, these researchers studied the influence, if any, of vitamin B_6 on somatomedin activity. They found that plasma somatomedin activity was reduced in laboratory rats administered a diet deficient in vitamin B_6 for four weeks. Their studies demonstrate that plasma growth hormone levels remain unchanged while the plasma insulin levels were markedly lowered. They conclude that the reduction in somatomedin activity appears to be associated with a factor that is not growth hormone–dependent. The reduction in somatomedin activity may be due to the lowered insulin levels or perhaps even related to an effect of vitamin B_6 deficiency itself.

This study demonstrates that the activities of one or more hormones may be altered or even modified by the presence or absence of one or more specific nutrients, in this case, vitamin B_6. While this work demonstrates a relationship between hormonal activity and vitamin B_6, the earlier work of Pfeiffer (1975) reports that vitamin B_6, along with the trace element zinc, is depleted as a result of stress exposure. Also, since these studies demonstrate a relationship between vitamin B_6, hormonal activity, and trace minerals, there may be relationships between other hormones and nutrients that are necessary for their optimal physiological activity.

As in the case of the other B vitamins described, and in view of the role vitamin B_6 plays in intermediate metabolism, the need for this vitamin may increase as metabolism is increased as a result of various types of stress exposure.

VITAMIN B_{12} (CYANOCOBALAMIN)

Vitamin B_{12} is commonly known as the "red vitamin." This name refers to its characteristic color. It is the only vitamin that contains a mineral substance, cobalt, that is essential for life. It is also unique because it is not found in any plants. Its dietary intake therefore depends on the amount of animal proteins that are consumed and absorbed by the body.

Vitamin B_{12} is stable in dry form but is destroyed upon contact with acid or alkaline solutions, alcohol, sleeping pills, and estrogen. It is unstable in the presence of light and may be affected by temperature changes. Small losses of the vitamin may occur under normal cooking conditions.

The presence of this vitamin is necessary for the adequate functioning of every cell in the body. It is a component of various coenzymes and is involved in the synthesis of nucleic acids; in particular, DNA synthesis. The vitamin also plays a role in carbohydrate and fat metabolism and possibly protein metabolism. In combination with folate (folic acid), vitamin B_{12} plays a role in maintaining the integrity of myelin in the nervous system. It is involved in nervous system metabolism. A lack of this vitamin can result in neurological damage. Vitamin B_{12} is essential for the formation of red blood cells. Therefore lack of it can result in pernicious anemia and perhaps other macrocytic anemias. Vitamin B_{12} can be used for both prophylaxis and treatment in these disorders.

Vitamin B_{12} is not assimilated very well unless calcium is present. Hence calcium is necessary for the vitamin to properly function in the body. The thyroid gland also plays a role in the proper functioning of vitamin B_{12}. Excess vitamin B_{12} is found in highest concentration in the liver, brain, heart, pancreas, bone marrow, and blood.

In general, cyanocobalamin will promote growth, maintain the integrity of the nervous system, improve mental alertness, relieve fatigue and irritability, increase energy, result in a more efficient use of protein, carbohydrates, and fats, and form and regenerate red blood cells.

Deficiency Disorders

A deficiency of vitamin B_{12} can result in serious disorders, among which are pernicious anemia (the most common disorder), neural cell dysfunction leading to brain damage, and possible epithelial cell alterations.

Since Americans consume a high protein diet, vitamin B_{12} deficiency is generally not commonly found in the United States. It is possible, however, that strict vegetarians, who have no animal food as part of their diet, may develop a lack of this vitamin. A diet that is low in vitamin B_1 and high in folic acid (characteristic of a vegetarian diet) may mask a deficiency of vitamin B_{12}. Sometimes it may take several years for a vitamin B_{12} deficiency to manifest itself.

Toxicity

There are no known toxic effects of this vitamin.

Vitamin B_{12}, Folic Acid, and Stress

The relationship of vitamin B_{12} and stress in laboratory animals has been studied. May et al. (1952) describe the effect of various stress conditions on the vitamin content of liver and the development of anemia in monkeys. The B vitamins in question are B_{12} and folic acid. The stress conditions are infection and inflammation. In stress conditions, vitamin B_{12} decreased from a control level of 1 microgram to a range of 0.8 microgram to 0.5 microgram while folic acid decreased from a control level of 1.10 microgram to a range of 0.62 to 0.3 microgram (1 microgram = one millionth of a gram). The data indicate that the stress of both infection and inflammation significantly reduced both liver folate and B_{12} levels. These researchers also found that a reduction in liver folate further induces the deficiency condition of megaloblastic anemia.

In humans, it appears that any type of chronic stress exposure in which metabolism is increased also increases the need for vitamin B_{12}. Vitamin B_{12} injections have been used for years in the alleviation of nervousness and fatigue. This may be related to the role vitamin B_{12} plays in the nervous system and perhaps in the red blood cells. Determination of a more specific role that vitamin B_{12} may play in the stress response awaits further investigative effort.

VITAMIN B$_{13}$ (OROTIC ACID)

Vitamin B$_{13}$ plays a role in the metabolism of folic acid and vitamin B$_{12}$. There is, however, little information available about this vitamin. Vitamin B$_{13}$ is not presently available in the United States but can be obtained in Europe. It is used in the treatment of multiple sclerosis.

Deficiency Disorders

Deficiency of this vitamin may lead to liver dysfunction. A deficiency of vitamin B$_{13}$ may lead to cell degeneration in patients suffering from multiple sclerosis.

Toxicity

There are no known toxic effects of this vitamin.

Vitamin B$_{13}$ and Stress

The relationship between this vitamin and the effect of stress are not yet clarified.

VITAMIN B$_{15}$ (PANGAMIC ACID)

Not much is known about vitamin B$_{15}$. Therefore, its essential nutritional requirement in humans has not yet been established. To date, it is not considered to be a vitamin in the true sense of the word. This substance has been researched and used by the Russians, and a description of its effects can be found in the Russian literature.

Basically, vitamin B$_{15}$ is an antioxidant and functions much like vitamin E. It aids in the prevention of tissue hypoxia (too low a level of oxygen). It plays a role in the metabolism of carbohydrates, fat, and proteins.

The Russians list several benefits for the use of this vitamin, among which are a stimulant for immune responsivity, a means of lowering blood levels of cholesterol, a combat for fatigue, and relief in the symptoms of angina, liver disease, diabetes, hypertension, and skin disorders. The Russians have also found it useful in treating autism, schizophrenia, and drug and alcoholic addiction.

Although research needs to be done on this substance, some evidence indicates that a deficiency may result in heart disease and a decreased amount of oxygen reaching tissues, resulting in long-term tissue damage.

Toxicity

There are no indications of any toxic effects produced by this vitamin.

Vitamin B_{15} and Stress

Russian athletes include vitamin B_{15} supplementation as part of their daily dietary intake. It has been reported in the Russian literature that vitamin B_{15} plays a role in decreasing muscle fatigue during certain types of exercise stress. The Russians report that a decrease in the level of lactic acid in the body may mediate this effect. In view of this, vitamin B_{15} may play a very important role in the elicitation of the stress response. However, further work needs to be done to clarify its physiological role in the body as well as its role in the elicitation of the stress response.

VITAMIN B_{17} (LAETRILE)

Vitamin B_{17} is a simple compound consisting of molecules of sugar, cyanide, and benzaldehyde. It occurs in nature in the pits of apricots. This vitamin has produced much controversy over its claimed specific cancer preventive properties. It is not accepted as a treatment of choice for cancer in the United States, although several states have legalized it and it is used legally in several countries throughout the world. Much literature is available on the use of laetrile in cancer treatment or prevention. If you are interested in this form of treatment approach, consultation with a physician knowledgeable in nutrition is highly recommended.

Deficiency Disorders

There are no known specific deficiency diseases associated with a lack of this vitamin. Perhaps a decreased resistance to certain types of cancer may occur as a result of a chronic vitamin B_{17} deficiency. Further research needs to be done to clarify the role played by this vitamin not only in cancer treatment but also its general physiological role in the body.

Toxicity

Levels of toxicity of this vitamin have not been established.

Vitamin B_{17} and Stress

There is no evidence to date to implicate this vitamin as playing a direct role in the stress response.

NIACIN (NICOTINIC ACID, NIACINAMIDE, NICOTINAMIDE)

Niacin (nicotinic acid) is another water-soluble vitamin belonging to the vitamin B complex family. It is a fairly stable substance in the presence of heat, acid, and alkaline solutions. The range of temperatures used in ordinary cooking does not generally destroy niacin, nor is it destroyed by oxidation. It is probably one of the most stable of the vitamins. It is chemically related to nicotine, but has very different physiological properties.

Niacin is found only in plants, but another substance, the amide of niacin called niacinamide, is found in animals.

The amino acid tryptophan, present in the body, allows the body to produce its own niacin. However, vitamins B_1, B_2, and B_6 must be present for the synthesis of niacin to occur from its precursor substance, tryptophan.

Niacin functions as a component of two coenzyme systems that play a role in tissue respiration and oxidation. In particular, niacin aids in the oxidation of carbohydrates.

Niacin is necessary for healthy brain function and for maintaining the integrity of the nervous system. It is thought to be necessary for the synthesis of several hormones of the endocrine system, such as the sex hormones, insulin, and cortisone. It is thought to play a role in maintaining a healthy gastrointestinal system. It helps to maintain healthy skin. Niacin is known to lower cholesterol levels, play a role in hydrochloric acid production, and participate in the metabolism of proteins, carbohydrates, and fats. Niacin aids in increasing the circulation and may reduce high blood pressure. In many instances, niacinamide rather than niacin is often used, since it does not cause the severe red flushing and itching of the skin that niacin itself may cause. The flush, caused by a generalized peripheral vasodilatation, is only temporary and generally disappears in a matter of minutes.

Deficiency Disorders

Niacin is stored in the liver. Since niacin is involved in the oxidation of carbohydrates, consuming large quantitites of sugars and starches will result in a deficiency of niacin in the body.

The deficiency disease of niacin is pellagra. It is characterized by several symptoms involving the skin, the brain, the nervous system, the gastrointestinal system, and the mucous membranes. Disturbances of the gastrointestinal tract may be manifested by a red swollen tongue, soreness in the mouth with possible canker sores, insomnia, and mental disorders such as depression, irritability, and anxiety. Possible impairment of memory, disorientation, and confusion may also result. The skin may become dry and scaly. Mucous membranes of the mouth and esophagus may become nonfunctional. Hydrochloric acid production may cease.

Recovery from pellagra occurs rapidly upon adequate administration of niacin. Human pellagra rarely exists without deficiencies in both vitamins B_1 and B_2. However, in the United States, pellagra is not common. Cases have been reported to occur among the elderly and chronic alcoholics. Secondary deficiencies have been reported in such conditions as chronic diarrhea and cirrhosis.

Toxicity

Niacin has been shown to be basically nontoxic. However, prolonged use may result in disturbances of the gastrointestinal tract.

Niacin and Stress

As has been described, several of the vitamins of the B complex family ameliorate or block the physiological effects of various types of stressors in both humans and animals.

The work of Hrubes and Benes (1967) and Benes and Hrubes (1968) describes the effect of nicotinic acid on changes in serum free fatty acids induced by stress in laboratory animals. Benes and Hrubes exposed two groups of rats to the stress exposure of intermittent electric shocks. By previous experimental criteria, one group possessed a good measure of stress adaptation and the other a low ability to adapt. These researchers found that as a result of stress exposure, the serum free fatty acid levels increased in both groups, but the animals with a low ability to adapt had a significantly higher level of free fatty acids. They found that nicotinic acid, at a dosage of 50 milligrams/kilogram, completely blocked the stress-induced increase in free fatty acid levels in both groups of rats.

Using half that dosage, they found that nicotinic acid blocked the stress effects only in the group of rats with greater stress adaptability.

In another investigation, Hrubes and Benes (1967) studied the time course of nicotinic acid on stress-induced changes in nonesterified fatty acids (NEFA) in rat serum. They subjected one group of rats to the stress of physical exertion and found a marked rise in NEFA. The rise was maintained for 30 minutes after the stress was removed. Rats pretreated with nicotinic acid did not show any rise in NEFA. Another group of rats was subjected to the emotional stress of intermittent electric shock for two hours. At the end of this stressful period, serum NEFA were markedly elevated and decreased back to control levels one hour after the termination of the stress exposure. In the group of rats undergoing the same stress exposure and pretreated with nicotinic acid, the elevation of NEFA was completely blocked. Hrubes and Benes found the blockade to be more complete in the emotionally stressed condition than in the case of physical exertion. Their work confirms the protective effect of nicotinic acid during both physical and emotional stress. The protective effect appears to be mediated through nicotinic acid's action in preventing the mobilization of NEFA from adipose tissue. Other researchers have observed this protective effect during stress exposure at different administering doses of nicotinic acid (Bombelli et al. 1965).

Several researchers have demonstrated that nicotinic acid appears to exert a protective effect by blocking the mobilization of free fatty acids from fat tissue in humans (Carlson et al. 1968; Carlson and Orö 1962; Carlson and Pernow 1959; Carlson et al. 1963). Carlson et al. (1968) subjected two groups of male volunteers and a control group to emotional stressors. One group received 3 grams of nicotinic acid in the early stages of the experiment while the other group did not receive nicotinic acid. Measurement of the stress response showed an increase in the levels of free fatty acids and triglycerides in arterial plasma, an increase in catecholamine excretion, an increase in heart rate, and an increase in both systolic and diastolic blood pressures. In the group treated with nicotinic acid, the stress-induced rise in free fatty acids was inhibited by nicotinic acid and the rise in triglycerides was reversed. On the other hand, nicotinic acid did not affect the stress-induced increases in catecholamine excretion, heart rate, and systolic and diastolic blood pressures. According to Carlson et al. (1968), the reduced response of free fatty acids as a result of emotional stress during nicotinic acid treatment implies a blockade or inhibition of the stress-induced enhancement of lipid mobilization.

Carlson has done other work to show that this blockade is a result of the inhibition of lipolysis occuring in adipose tissue (Carlson 1963; Carlson 1965). Along with others (Carlson et al. 1965), Carlson has also explored the implications of these findings in relation to cardiovascular disease, since there have been several cases reported of elevated plasma levels of triglycerides in patients with coronary heart disease.

In certain reported cases, nicotinic acid in massive doses (3 grams or more) has been administered to patients with hypercholesterolemia (Altschul 1965) and has also been administered to patients suffering certain types of mental illness (Hoffer 1963). In many of these cases, the result has been an alleviation of symptoms.

FOLIC ACID (FOLACIN, FOLATE)

Folic acid is a yellow crystalline substance that is easily destroyed when exposed to heat (cooking), light, and neutral and alkaline solutions. It is stable in acid media and sparingly soluble in water.

Folic acid can be readily absorbed from the small intestine. When it is present in excess amounts in the body, it is stored in the liver.

Folic acid works in conjunction with vitamin B_{12}. Both vitamins are interdependent and both are necessary for the manufacture of some of the essential components of red blood cells. Folic acid is used in the treatment of pernicious anemia, macrocytic anemia, and sprue. The major role of this vitamin is in the prevention of megaloblastic anemia in humans.

This vitamin is also necessary for the synthesis of the nucleic acids, RNA and DNA. Both of these substances are necessary for cellular growth and reproduction. Folic acid plays an important role in protein metabolism and in the use of carbohydrates.

Deficiency Disorders

The main folic acid deficiency disease is severe megaloblastic anemia. This can be seen more among the poorer populations in the tropics than among the more affluent societies. There is some evidence to indicate that a folate deficiency leads to a decrease in immunosuppression (Guss et al. 1975). Folic acid deficiency can occur quite commonly during pregnancy, especially during the last trimester, when the need for it is definitely increased. Also, many gastrointestinal disturbances can reduce the absorption of folic acid, leading to a condition of secondary folic acid deficiency.

Many drugs may interfere with the absorption of folacin. Ascorbic acid, oral contraceptives, and several of the anticonvulsant drugs used in the treatment of epilepsy are known to lead to decreased serum levels of folacin. Drugs used in the treatment of tumor malignancies may also be included in this category. There is evidence that chronic alcoholism influences the metabolism of folic acid and could thereby result in folic acid deficiency.

Toxicity

There are no known toxic effects reported concerning this vitamin.

Folacin and Stress

The role that folic acid plays in relation to stress has not been clearly elucidated.

BIOTIN (COENZYME R, VITAMIN H)

Biotin was formally designated vitamin H but has since been categorized with the B complex vitamins. It is a very active physiological substance. In small doses, it can have a marked influence on the growth of yeast and other micoorganisms. In fact, it is considered to be a potent yeast growth factor.

Biotin is stable in the presence of heat and light but unstable in the presence of oxidation and alkaline solutions. Raw egg white contains a protein called avidin. This substance is antagonistic to biotin and therefore prevents its absorption. Cooking the eggs destroys the antagonistic effect of avidin on biotin since the avidin is denatured, thus liberating the biotin.

Biotin plays an important role in many of the chemical reactions that take place in the body. It participates in the synthesis of ascorbic acid and acts as a coenzyme in the normal metabolism of proteins, carbohydrates, and fats. Folic acid is vital for lipid synthesis in the body.

Biotin also acts synergistically with vitamins A_1, B_2, B_6, and niacin in the maintenance of healthy skin. It helps in the body's use of protein, vitamins B_5, B_{12}, and folic acid.

Deficiency Disorders

Since biotin is found in a wide variety of foods and is synthesized by the intestinal flora, a deficiency is not very common. A deficiency can occur if unusually large amounts of raw egg whites are consumed. Some deficiency symptoms are depression, exhaustion, muscle pain, dry skin, and impairment of fat metabolism. Overall lipid metabolism may be severely compromised in severe states of biotin deficiency.

Toxicity

Biotin has not been reported to result in any toxic effects.

Biotin and Stress

The role that biotin plays in relation to stress has not been clearly elucidated.

CHOLINE

Choline is classified as a member of the B complex vitamins. It is widely distributed in plant and animal tissues. It is lipotropic; that is, it aids the body in the use of cholesterol and fats. Choline is a component of lecithin and other phospholipids and acts in conjunction with inositol in participating in fat metabolism. Choline also participates in protein and carbohydrate metabolism.

Choline has the ability to penetrate the blood-brain barrier, and therefore it penetrates brain tissue. It belongs to a class of substances known as amines and is a precursor in the synthesis of acetylcholine, which is an important neurotransmitter substance that is found in the brain and in the nervous system. Therefore choline is also an important chemical substance involved in nerve transmission. In particular, it is involved in nerve transmission in those regions of the brain associated with memory.

Choline appears to emulsify cholesterol, thereby preventing its accumulation along the arterial walls of the vasculature. It is therefore helpful in preventing atherosclerosis, hardening of the arteries, and high circulating cholesterol levels. Choline has been successful in the treatment of insomnia, some visual disturbances, and high blood pressure. It has also been useful in the treatment of fatty livers in chronic alcoholics.

Deficiency Disorders

A deficiency of choline may result in hardening of the arteries, cirrhosis and fatty degeneration of the liver, impaired kidney function, and ulcers.

Toxicity

Toxic effects of choline are not presently known.

Choline and Stress

The role that choline plays in relation to the elicitation of the stress response has not been clearly elucidated.

INOSITOL

Inositol is a member of the B complex vitamin family. It is an integral constituent of the brain, kidney, liver, heart, and skeletal muscles. In combination with choline, it aids in the synthesis of lecithin, a phospholipid found in several animal tissues and necessary for the removal of fats from liver. Like choline, it plays a role in the metabolism of fats and cholesterol and it aids in the lowering of blood cholesterol levels. Inositol also helps in the growth of hair and in the prevention of eczema.

Deficiency Disorders

The deficiency of inositol in animals results in the loss of hair, growth retardation, and eye defects. Some possible deficiencies in humans are atherosclerosis, baldness, high cholesterol levels, excess body weight, heart disease and eczema.

Toxicity

There are no known toxic effects associated with inositol.

Inositol and Stress

The role that inositol plays in relation to stress has not been clearly elucidated.

para-AMINOBENZOIC ACID (PABA)

PABA is a member of the B complex vitamin family and it can be synthesized in the body. As a component of folic acid, it participates in its synthesis. In conjunction with pantothenic acid, PABA was found to restore gray hair to its natural color in animal experimentation. PABA is also known for its effectiveness in sunscreening. As a coenzyme, it is involved in the use of proteins. It is important for maintaining the integrity of the intestinal tract.

This vitamin is used in the treatment of arthritis, gout, various skin disorders, rheumatic fever, baldness, graying hair, and possibly stress. It can aid in keeping the skin healthy and wrinkle free.

Deficiency Disorders

Eczema, depression, fatigue, and digestive disorders are some of the deficiency symptoms associated with a lack of PABA in the body.

Toxicity

There are no known toxic effects associated with PABA.

PABA and Stress

The role that PABA plays in relation to stress has not been clearly elucidated.

OTHER B VITAMINS

Other B vitamins exist and play a major role in animal species other than humans. For example, it is thought that vitamin B_3 is important in chick nutrition while vitamin B_4 is necessary in rat and possibly chick nutrition. Vitamin B_4 is thought to consist of a combination of the amino acids arginine, cysteine, and glycine. It helps prevent weakness of the muscles. The designations B_3 and B_4 are no longer used to name members of the vitamin B complex family.

Originally named in error, vitamins B_7, B_8, and B_9 are not presently designated as substances belonging to the B complex family.

Vitamins B_{10} and B_{11} were names given to substances now known to be a mixture of folic acid and vitamin B_{12}.

Vitamin B_{14} is a term used to describe a substance that has been isolated from human urine. It is not at present considered to be an important B complex vitamin for humans. When this substance is placed in bone-marrow cultures, it appears to strongly influence cell-proliferating activity. However, when placed in the presence of certain suspensions of neoplastic cells, it appears to exert an inhibitory effect.

VITAMIN F (UNSATURATED FATTY ACIDS, ARACHIDONIC ACID, LINOLEIC ACID, LINOLENIC ACID)

Vitamin F is a formerly used term for essential fatty acids. It is composed of the essential unsaturated fatty acids obtained from various types of foodstuffs. This vitamin is, of course, soluble in fats and aids in the promotion of saturated fat oxidation. It is unstable in the presence of heat and oxygen.

The substances that constitute vitamin F can help in preventing the buildup of cholesterol deposits in the walls of the arterial bed. They play a role in the growth of the organism and influence glandular activity. They may aid in maintaining healthy skin and hair. These substances may also be effective in a program of weight reduction since they are involved in the oxidation of saturated fats.

Deficiency Disorders

A possible deficiency disorder due to lack of vitamin F is eczema.

Toxicity

There are no known toxic effects of these essential fatty acids, although when taken in excess they may lead to an increase in weight.

VITAMIN G

This is an obsolete name for riboflavin, which is now known as vitamin B_2.

VITAMIN H

This is an obsolete name for biotin.

VITAMIN H^1

This is another name for *para*-aminobenzoic acid.

VITAMIN L

This is a vitamin that is found to be necessary for the process of lactation in rats.

VITAMIN M

This is an obsolete name for folic acid.

VITAMIN P
(CITRUS BIOFLAVONOIDS, HESPERIDIN, RUTIN, C COMPLEX)

These substances are associated with vitamin C and are found widely distributed in nature as pigments in fruits, vegetables, and flowers. Their presence is thought to be necessary for the proper absorption of vitamin C in the body. The flavonoids are also included in this group and are the substances that supply the yellow and orange color to citrus fruits.

Vitamin P stands for a permeability factor. This group of substances are necessary for the normal integrity of capillary membranes and for normal membrane permeability. They act basically to strengthen the capillary walls, thereby making them less fragile, less susceptible to bruising and more able to protect against infection. Vitamin P, therefore, helps to prevent ruptures and hemorrhages in capillaries. In the strict sense of the word, vitamin P is not considered to be a vitamin. These substances work synergistically with vitamin C and increase its effectiveness. They aid vitamin C in maintaining the health of the connective tissues of the body. Bioflavonoids given to athletes accelerate the healing process involved in muscle and joint injuries.

Deficiency Disorders

The major deficiency disorder associated with a lack of bioflavonoids in the body is a fragility of the capillary walls.

Toxicity

There are no known toxic effects associated with vitamin P.

VITAMIN P-P

This is the name given to a pellagra-preventing factor. It is now known as niacinamide, a member of the B complex family.

VITAMIN T

There is little known about this substance and no supplements for human consumption are yet on the market. It appears to play a role in the formation of blood platelets and blood coagulation. It may be beneficial in the prevention and treatment of certain anemias and hemophilia.

Toxicity

To date, no known toxic effects exist for this substance.

VITAMIN U (CABAGIN, ANTIULCER VITAMIN)

Not much is known about this vitamin. It is thought to be necessary for the growth of chicks. It appears to be strongly involved in the healing of ulcers although much investigative work needs to be done in this area.

The vitamin is found in raw cabbage, from which it derives its name.

Toxicity

No known toxic effects exist for this substance.

5

THE MICRO MINERAL ELEMENTS

INTRODUCTION

A mineral is either an inorganic element or compound that is found in nature and is generally in the solid state. It is found in the ground and is not of plant or animal origin. Plants derive their mineral substances from the ground. Animals derive their minerals from the plants they eat, which have previously drawn the minerals from the ground. Humans, in turn, obtain minerals directly from plants or from animals that have previously eaten the plants.

Minerals can be viewed as being essential raw materials necessary for life, for mental and physical well-being. Their presence in the body, in adequate amounts, is absolutely necessary for the maintenance of human health. All the tissues and fluids of the body contain various amounts of minerals. The body itself is composed of approximately 5 percent minerals. Today, minerals are considered to be just as important as vitamins, if not more so. Although the body can manufacture some vitamins for itself, it is basically dependent on outside sources for most of its vitamins and all of its minerals.

The minerals necessary for normal body function are present in small amounts in the body, hence minerals are generally referred to as micronutrients. Mineral elements present in the body in extremely small amounts—less than 0.005 percent—are referred to as trace elements. As with the vitamins, there are some minerals that do not as yet have an accepted well-defined or established human requirement even though some investigative work indicates that they may be physiologically active in specific cases.

More than 20 different minerals, both metals and nonmetals, are thought to be vital to the maintenance of human health. The possibility exists, however, that more minerals may be added to this list.

Minerals play several vital roles in the body. Like the vitamins, they do not supply any calories. Some of the important physiological activities in which minerals actively participate in the body are listed below.

- Minerals form the essential ingredients of every living cell. For example, the mineral phosphorus is found in both the nucleus and cytoplasm of every cell. Minerals, at the cellular level, participate in the vital processes of growth, oxidation, and secretion.
- Minerals form essential components in various enzyme systems involved in metabolism and hormone synthesis.
- Minerals are important for nerve transmission. For example, if minerals such as sodium, potassium, calcium, magnesium, and in some cases, chloride, are not present in the right concentrations in the fluids bathing the nerve cells, nerve transmission may be interfered with.
- In a similar manner, minerals regulate the excitability (contraction) of muscle cells.
- Minerals regulate not only the permeability of nerve and muscle cell membranes, but of cell membranes in general, including capillary vessels.
- Minerals form a large part of the more solid structures of the body, such as bones, teeth, and nails. The minerals calcium, phosphorus, and magnesium are essential components of the structure of bones and teeth.
- Minerals are necessary for the maintenance of proper acid-base balance.
- Minerals play an important role in regulating the appropriate movement of intracellular and extracellular body fluids so as to maintain equilibrium across the cells. Also, certain minerals—sodium, for example—contribute to water and electrolyte balance. Hence minerals play an important role in the regulation of blood volume.
- Many of the minerals form an integral part of the structure of many organs or tissues of the body. For example, iodine is found in the thyroid gland; copper and iron are found in the liver and other tissues; iron, iodine, and fluorine form an essential constituent of red blood cells and are necessary for the synthesis of hemoglobin; and chlorine is found in hydrochloric acid, as well as in some other gastric juices.

- Minerals are essential components of the secretions of many glands, both endocrine and exocrine.
- Minerals play a role as catalysts in several important biochemical reactions. For example, the presence of zinc is necessary for insulin synthesis. The proper intestinal absorption of vitamin B_{12} occurs in the presence of calcium.

As with other families of substances in the body, minerals generally do not function alone. A familiar example is that of calcium and phosphorus, which exist together in a definite ratio in bone. No mineral acts in isolation, just as no hormone acts alone. Several of the vitamins act synergistically. Several interrelationships exist among the minerals in the body, all of which contribute toward balance and homeostasis in the maintenance of health.

Approximately 20 to 30 grams of mineral salts along with 2 to 3 liters of water are excreted from the body daily. These mineral salts must necessarily be replaced daily through the diet. The basic dietary recommended requirements for some of the minerals have been established. Other minerals exist in such small concentrations in biological fluids that it has been difficult not only to assign a recommended dietary requirement for them but also to assign them a definite physiological role. Many of the mineral elements play indirect roles. For example, in the treatment of pernicious anemia, the trace element cobalt is necessary but not effective when it acts alone. Cobalt forms an essential part of the structure of vitamin B_{12} which is effective in the treatment of the disorder.

The human body is composed of the following mineral elements in micro amounts: calcium, phosphorus, potassium, sulfur, sodium, chloride, magnesium, and silicon. The body is also composed of elements that are present in smaller, trace amounts (generally less than 0.01 percent). These trace elements, which have an important physiological function, include arsenic, barium, boron, bromine, chromium, cobalt, copper, fluorine, iodine, iron, manganese, molybdenum, rubidium, selenium, strontium, vanadium, and zinc.

Trace elements whose physiological functions have not been clearly defined include aluminum, antimony, gallium, lithium, nickel, silver, tin, and titanium. If present in excess quantities aluminum, cadmium, fluorine, lead, mercury, and vanadium produce a variety of toxic effects. Elements known to exhibit toxic effects but whose physiological function have not been clearly defined include beryllium, bismuth, and bromine.

These elements collectively are referred to as the toxic elements. In particular, beryllium, cadmium, lead, and mercury are metals that are products of industrialization. These mineral elements are considered to be hazardous to human health.

A summary of the source and the U.S. Recommended Daily Allowances for some of these minerals is presented in Table A-II of the Appendix.

In addition to the material presented in this and the next two chapters, the reader is referred to the more comprehensive work of Beisel and Pekarek (1972) concerning the effects of acute stress and trace mineral element metabolism, the work of Rosenberg and Solomons (1984) concerning mineral nutrient absorption and malabsorption, and the work of Prasad (1982) concerning the clinical, biochemical, and nutritional aspects of the trace mineral elements.

CALCIUM

Calcium is the most prevalent mineral element found in the body. It functions, along with phosphorus, to maintain healthy bones and teeth. Ninety-nine percent of all the calcium found in the body resides in the bones. The rest is in cells and in extracellular fluids and is very important in the regulation of such processes as cell membrane permeability, excitation-contraction coupling in muscle, and nerve transmission.

Calcium works in conjunction with magnesium to maintain the health of the cardiovascular system. It plays an important role in the clotting mechanism of whole blood. Calcium plays a role in certain enzyme systems of the body involved in hormone secretory activity and in certain metabolic processes. It appears to act as a regulator of other mineral elements, vitamins, and hormones in the body. For example, adequate amounts of calcium aid the body in better using iron and vitamin D. Calcium appears to play a corrective role with sodium, potassium, and magnesium, should these elements be present in greater than normal amounts. Calcium is necessary for the proper functioning of the parathyroid hormone. Obviously, the importance of calcium in the body cannot be overestimated.

Calcium is absorbed into the bloodstream from the small intestine, a process that depends on a number of factors. The most important are the availability of vitamin D and the degree of acidity of the digestive fluids. Both vitamin D and a more acid or low pH environment in the intestine directly enhance the calcium absorption process.

Some substances can restrict calcium absorption should this element be present in larger than normal amounts. Such substances include oxalic acid (found in tea, cocoa, chocolate, spinach, soybeans, and rhubarb), phytic acid (found in certain cereals), and too high a level of phosphorus or phosphorous compounds. These substances can combine with calcium to form a calcium phosphate compound, which cannot be absorbed easily by the body. However, adequate or generous amounts of calcium in the diet can override this interference effect and calcium absorption need not be compromised.

Blood levels of calcium and phosphorus are regulated by para-thyroid hormone (parathormone), secreted by the parathyroid gland. This hormone influences the blood levels of calcium and phosphorus through its influence on bone, intestines, and kidney. Parathyroid hormone acts directly on bone to increase the blood levels of calcium and phosphorus by promoting bone reabsorption. It acts on the intestines by promoting the absorption of calcium and phosphorus into the blood and it acts on the kidney by enhancing calcium reabsorption and increasing phosphate excretion. Parathyroid hormone and calcium interact with each other in a feedback mechanism. Increased levels of parathyroid hormone enhance calcium blood levels. As blood levels of calcium rise, parathyroid hormone secretion is depressed. When blood calcium levels are depressed, parathyroid hormone secretion is increased to again raise blood calcium levels to normal.

Another hormone, called calcitonin (thyrocalcitonin), secreted by the thyroid gland, also regulates blood levels of calcium. Calcitonin influences bone tissue, which results in a release of calcium into the bloodstream. Calcitonin acts reciprocally to parathyroid hormone, and its secretion is also thought to be influenced by calcium blood levels.

As blood levels of calcium decrease calcitonin secretion is decreased, and as blood levels of calcium increase calcitonin secretion is increased, which, in turn, lowers blood calcium concentration. Calcitonin is therefore a calcium-lowering hormone while parathyroid hormone is calcium-increasing. Factors such as dietary intake and metabolism, among others, contribute to maintaining the plasma levels of calcium and phosphorous within the normal physiological range.

Deficiency Conditions

Lack of calcium can slow growth in children and in extreme cases can result in rickets in children and osteomalacia or osteoporosis in adults. Rickets and osteomalacia are generally accompanied by a lack of phosphorus and vitamin D. Osteoporosis is more common in older people. The bones become very brittle and fragile due to a decrease in the supply of calcium and protein in the body. Osteoporosis can cause weakness and is often painful. It can result in a shrinking of the total mass of bone. Some people may actually shrink in height as they grow older. Osteoporosis can be caused by the long-term use of such drugs as cortisone, which can result in the loss of calcium by the body. Osteoporosis may also be linked to a decrease in estrogen. A decrease in estrogen production and calcium loss in postmenopausal women appear to be related. The incidence of osteoporosis is known to be greater in postmenopausal women.

The development of teeth in early childhood may be retarded by low calcium levels, and periodontal disease may also occur.

Calcium deficiency may occur during or after recovery from a serious illness, surgery, or infectious disease, all of which require extra calcium and other nutrients to expedite the recovery process. In such states, gastrointestinal absorption may be somewhat impaired and therefore calcium absorption may be severely restricted. Increased amounts of calcium can offset this type of interference.

Other conditions of calcium deficiency include the development of nerve-muscle symptomology, such as feelings of fatigue, muscle twitching, muscle cramping, and nerve and muscle spasms.

When the body is not receiving enough exercise, more calcium is needed. If a person is confined to bed even for a few days, an increased amount of calcium is lost (approximately 200 milligrams per day or so). This added loss of calcium should be replaced by dietary supplementation above the normal required intake of calcium. In general, growing children and pregnant and lactating women have higher than normal calcium needs. Emotional and other types of stress also result in a loss of calcium by the body.

PHOSPHORUS

Phosphorus is another mineral element that is found in every cell and is involved in several chemical reactions throughout the body. While phosphorus functions alone in many instances, it also works in conjunction with calcium. Calcium and phosphorus must exist in a definite ratio and this ratio must be maintained. The ratio for the two minerals to work effectively is 2.5 to 1 or 2 to 1.

About 70 to 80 percent of the phosphorus present in the body is found combined with calcium in bones and teeth, about 10 percent is found in muscle, and a much smaller percentage is found in nerve tissue.

Both calcium and phosphorus are important and necessary for the process of nerve stimulation and muscle contraction.

Phosphorus is present in proteins, carbohydrates, and fats, and by itself it plays an important role in certain metabolic processes involving all of these nutrients and energy production. For example, phosphorus compounds such as adenosine triphosphate (ATP) and phosphocreatine are the main sources of energy production in muscle contraction.

Phosphorus is an essential constituent of nucleic acids and the nucleoproteins that participate in the transference of inherited characteristics during cell division. Vitamin D is important for the absorption and metabolism of phosphate by the body. Many of the B vitamins can function effectively only when they are combined with phosphorus. For example, niacin cannot be assimilated by the body unless it is combined with phosphorus.

Phosphorus is present in a wide variety of foodstuffs, so the possibility of a phosphorus deficiency in the diet becomes highly improbable. The richest food sources for both phosphorus and calcium are dairy products, eggs, meat, and fish. Phosphorus is present in the diet if a lot of processed foods are eaten. It is necessary to be aware of this, since a balance between calcium and phosphorus must be maintained in the body. Also, the aging process may result in decreased phosphorus and less calcium in the body, thus upsetting the necessary ratio that must exist between the two. Therefore, as we get older, it may be advisable to include extra calcium-containing foods in the diet.

Deficiency Conditions

A deficiency of phosphorus could result in a weakening of the bones, since the body will absorb this needed mineral from bones when it is not present in sufficient amounts in the body. Imperfect bone and teeth development, slowing of the growth process, rickets, and overall weakness are symptomatic of a phosphorus deficiency.

Calcium, Phosphorus, and Stress

Various types of stress exposure may influence the blood levels of calcium and phosphorus directly rather than having a direct effect on the hormones that influence these two elements. Research describes the effects of various types of stress exposure on the blood levels of calcium and phosphorous in both animals and humans. Newell and Beauchene (1975) present evidence that demonstrates that acid stress tends to decrease both serum calcium and phosphorus levels along with significant increases in the excretion of urinary total acid, calcium, and phosphorus in laboratory rats. Adler et al. (1968) have reported similar responses to acid stress in humans.

Some researchers report lowered levels of serum calcium in laboratory animals exposed to restraint stress (Hofmann et al 1979; Schwille et al. 1965; Schwille et al. 1974). Hofmann et al. discuss the influence of restraint stress on serum levels of calcium and phosphate in laboratory rats that were either left intact or thyroidectomized. These researchers found a significant stress-induced decrease in both total calcium and ionized calcium in the intact group but not in the thyroidectomized (calcitonin-absent) animals. In both groups of animals, they report a hyperphosphatemia (phosphate elevation in the blood) as a result of the stress exposure. Hofmann et al. suggest that hypocalcemia and hyperphosphatemia may be added to the list of symptoms associated with restraint stress in rats. While they found an increase of calcium efflux from bone, which would add calcium to the bloodstream, they infer that further studies involving parathyroid hormone secretory rates, histamine activity, catecholamine activity in the circulation, and other substances as well would add to our knowledge.

Other researchers report a decrease in serum phosphorus (hypophosphatemia) in subjects under heat stress (hyperthermia) (Iampietro et al 1961; and Coburn et al. 1966). A significant decrease in serum phosphorus was observed in sheep after transportation stress (Tollersrud et al. 1971).

Flynn et al. (1971) studied the correlation, if any, of certain mineral elements and adenohypophyseal adrenal cortical function (ACTH production) and stress. The adenohypophyseal adrenal cortical axis is activated as a result of almost all types of stress exposures. These researchers studied the involvement of some of the trace elements, including calcium, in the stress-induced activation of hypophyseal adrenal cortical axis in laboratory rats during the stress of hypotension. They found serum calcium to decrease slightly during stress and reach close to control levels upon recovery from stress. They therefore found little correlation between ACTH and calcium as a result of the stress of hypotension.

Tigranian et al. (1980) studied the levels of several hormones, electrolytes, and nutrients before and immediately after an academic examination in 15 male students and found the preexamination level of calcium and parathyroid hormone to be either increased or at the upper normal limit. The postexamination period showed no significant change in parathyroid hormone level while the increase in calcium was significant.

Rabie and Radulovacki (1971) studied the calcium content of cerebrospinal fluid in experimentally excited unanesthetized cats and found that the calcium concentration increased significantly following the period of excitation. It has been previously observed that after a latent period, sleep occurs for several hours in animals injected with calcium. Rabie and Radulovacki suggest that the stress-induced cerebrospinal fluid calcium rise may be part of a homeostatic mechanism within the brain itself that contributes to the maintenance of a quiet or nonexcited state for the animal before the onset of excitation. Among other possibilities, they suggest that such stress hormones as the catecholamines and ACTH may play a role in altering membrane permeability to calcium, thereby allowing an increased entry of calcium into the cerebrospinal fluid. They found no significant change in sodium and potassium levels before and after excitation.

Other researchers have studied the effect of stress on calcium uptake in the pituitary gland and brain of laboratory animals. Sabbot and Costin (1974b) subjected rats to cold stress exposure and found an increase in the uptake of calcium in the pituitary gland and certain regions of the brain. They found that cold stress induces a change in membrane permeability for calcium entry into the blood-brain and blood-pituitary barriers. Sabbot and Costin suggest a possible relationship between the secretion of hypothalamic and pituitary hormones, perhaps growth hormone releasing factor and ACTH or other stress hormones, and an increase in calcium uptake by the pituitary gland and brain.

In summary, it appears that various types of stress exposure result in a transient increase in the blood levels of both calcium and phosphorus. The increase in blood levels of calcium may be the result of a stress-induced calcium efflux from cells. Subsequently, both blood calcium and phosphorus levels are reduced. The stress-induced changes in phosphorus may be related to the changes occurring in calcium levels as a result of stress. Therefore, the overall effect of stress on these two mineral elements appears to be a lowering of both body calcium and phosphorus.

MAGNESIUM

Magnesium is a major mineral element that exists in all cells of the body. It is also one of the major cations (positive ions) found in the body. It serves as an activator or "starter" for many enzyme systems responsible for energy conversion. It is found in bones, muscles, soft tissue, and fluids bathing the cells. It also exists in the cerebrospinal fluid, plasma, and sweat. It is vital for the processes of excitation-contraction coupling in muscle, nerve transmission, and the synthesis of various essential cellular components.

The adult human contains approximately 21 to 28 grams of magnesium. It is the second most abundant cation in soft tissue after potassium. It maintains a ratio with potassium of about 1 to 5 or 1 to 6.

Magnesium is necessary for the metabolism and proper function of calcium, phosphorus, sodium, potassium, vitamin C, vitamin D, and parathyroid hormone.

Magnesium helps in the prevention of an excess buildup of calcium deposits in the body. Such deposits can result in gallstones and kidney stones.

Magnesium may aid in relieving nervous depression. It may play a role in the process of digestion.

Magnesium is an essential component in many enzymatic reactions in the body, particularly in reactions that generate high energy phosphate bonds, and it plays an important role in DNA synthesis and degradation.

Magnesium may play a role in promoting a healthy cardiovascular system. Various studies have shown that heart attack victims have less magnesium in their heart muscle than those who died from other causes. It has also been shown that there are fewer deaths from heart disease in regions where magnesium is in higher concentrations in the drinking water. However, more investigative work is necessary to provide conclusive proof of the interrelationships that may exist between magnesium and the health of the cardiovascular system.

Deficiency Conditions

The concentration of magnesium inside the cells is approximately 5 to 10 times its concentration in the blood, depending on the tissue studied. If magnesium leaves the cells, a transient increase in magnesium blood levels or a transient hypermagnesemia will result. Over a period of time, a negative magnesium balance will ensue as magnesium is continually lost from the cells and from the body. A state of magnesium deficiency can result. Low magnesium dietary intake will, of course, increase the probability of the onset of such a state. A negative magnesium balance can lead to an increased risk of cardiovascular disease. In both humans and animals, a causal relationship appears to exist between magnesium deficiency and myocardial disease.

Magnesium deficiency may also occur during the course of an illness. Diseases that may be associated with a magnesium deficiency are diabetes, alcoholism, gastrointestinal disorders, infections, and disorders of the thyroid and parathyroid glands. Also, various conditions of stress can result in a magnesium deficiency. Magnesium has often been termed an antistress mineral.

Some symptoms of magnesium defiency are muscle and nerve spasticity, convulsions, arrhythmia, and tachycardia.

Magnesium and Stress

Several studies indicate that stress exposure, both acute and chronic, can lead to magnesium deficiency.

Classen et al. (1971) exposed cats to the acute stress of blood withdrawal, catecholamine infusions, and asphyxia. An immediate increase in blood magnesium was found. This may be the result of a stress-induced cellular magnesium efflux, thus causing a transient hypermagnesemia. From these experiments one can infer that cells lose magnesium under stressful conditions. The loss of magnesium by the cells can lead to a negative magnesium balance, that is, a loss of body magnesium. Therefore these researchers suggest that sufficient amounts of magnesium should be part of the diet, particularly in individuals under chronic stress exposure. Classen et al. also conclude that a diet deficient in magnesium can sensitize the cells to fatal stress reactions.

In another published work, Classen (1981) states that from all reported data on animal and human studies, it appears justified to assume that human reactivity to various types of stress exposures can be aggravated by states of magnesium deficiency.

Other researchers have studied the magnesium content of the central nervous system (Chutkow 1972; Woodward and Reed 1969; Himly and Somjen 1968; Sabbot and Costin 1974a, 1974b). Sabbot and Costin studied the effect of cold stress on the uptake and distribution of calcium and magnesium in the rat brain and pituitary. They found that cold stress induced an increase in calcium uptake in the cortex, hippocampus, cerebellum, medulla, and pituitary gland. On the other hand, the uptake of magnesium by the cortex, hippocampus, and the pituitary gland was increased during cold stress. They found the uptake of calcium and magnesium to differ in the cortex and the hippocampus. The magnesium uptake levels were higher in the cortex than in the hippocampus while the opposite was true for calcium. These researchers conclude that cold stress induces changes in membrane permeability for both the blood-pituitary and blood-brain barriers for magnesium (Sabbot and Costin 1974a). This result is similar to previous findings on the stress-induced alteration in membrane permeability for calcium (Sabbot and Costin 1974b).

Günther et al. (1978) studied the effect of noise stress and magnesium deficiency in laboratory animals and found a synergistic effect between them. Ising (1981) also studied the interaction of noise stress and alterations in body magnesium in both animals and humans. From this study, Ising concludes that prolonged stress, together with marginal magnesium dietary intake, can result in a decrease in intracellular magnesium along with parallel increases in cellular calcium. Similarly, Raab et al. (1968) report an increase in myocardial calcium and a decrease in myocardial magnesium in laboratory rats during isolation stress.

Heroux et al. (1977), in their studies with experimental animals, demonstrate that a state of magnesium deficiency can in the long term compromise homeostasis. They show that this state is characterized by few overt deficiency symptoms. They suggest that a reduced resistance to stress as a result of magnesium deficiency, which may occur as a result of low dietary levels of magnesium over time, and which may not be associated with any manifest symptoms, may predispose humans to ischemic heart diesease.

B.M. Altura (1979), B.T. Altura (1980), and Altura and Altura (1974, 1978, 1981) studied the relationship between magnesium, vascular smooth muscle, and the cardiovascular system. B.T. Altura (1980) discusses the epidemiological evidence implicating magnesium deficiency in heart disease. This researcher reports that during decreased amounts of magnesium in the extracellular fluids, the blood vessels undergo sustained increases in tone and become more sensitive to constriction by circulating vasoactive agents. This is brought about possibly by an enhanced calcium influx. Altura proposes that a personality exhibiting Type A behavior (personality characterized by almost constant self-imposed stress) is compatible with an intermittent virtual magnesium deficiency, which could lead, in the long term, to coronary vasospasm, ischemia of the myocardium, and possibly heart tissue necrosis. Other researchers also report a deficiency in magnesium in relation to ischemic heart disease (Seelig 1974; Turlapaty and Altura 1980; Leary and Reyes 1983). Leary and Reyes present evidence that stress potentiates a state of magnesium deficiency. They also present experimental evidence indicating that a reduction in plasma magnesium levels may be associated with arterial spasms. Previously, Altura and Altura (1981) demonstrated in studies dealing with experimental animals that alterations in magnesium metabolism may have profound effects on the contractile state of vascular smooth muscle, which in turn could influence blood pressure.

Diuretics, particularly the thiazides, which are generally given in the treatment of hypertension, can enhance magnesium loss from the body. Dyckner and Wester (1983) studied the effect of magnesium on blood pressure. They administered magnesium supplements to 20 patients receiving long-term diuretic treatment for arterial hypertension or congestive heart failure. They report that both systolic and diastolic pressures decreased significantly with magnesium supplementation (in addition to the thiazide effects on blood pressure). They suggest that magnesium supplementation should be considered, at least as an additional treatment, in patients with arterial hypertension already maintained on a diuretic regimen.

Magnesium also may be lost from the body through the excessive use of laxatives and alcohol.

Cortisol secreted in response to enhanced levels of ACTH is elevated in the circulation as a result of practically all types of stress exposure. Flynn et al. (1971), in their studies of the mineral elements, observed little correlation between the stress-induced secretion of ACTH and magnesium.

Another point to consider is that most types of stressful stimuli induce an elevation in free fatty acid levels (Reynaert et al. 1976). This elevation has recently been demonstrated to decrease the free ionized levels of blood magnesium (Altura 1980). Stress-induced catecholamine release may also contribute to magnesium depletion. As mentioned previously, the possibility exists that as a result of the elicitation of the stress response there is an efflux of magnesium from the intracellular compartment which causes a transient hypermagnesemia, as observed by some researchers. But due to the presence of the stress-induced release of catecholamines and perhaps even free fatty acids, there is a subsequent loss of magnesium from the body (hypermagnesemauria) leading to decreased levels of plasma magnesium (hypomagnesemia).

In summary, there are many factors to consider with regard to the epidemiological and clinical studies available that relate hypomagnesemia or a state of magnesium deficiency to the chronic elicitation of the stress response, hypertension, cardiovascular damage, and death. The positive effects of magnesium supplementation in patients at risk have been indicated.

Magnesium metabolism has been shown to be influenced by several types of physical stress exposure. The stress of trauma and shock appear to elevate serum magnesium. This may occur as a consequence of a reduction in magnesium excretion and a release of magnesium from damaged and affected tissue. The stress of severe burns may result in a hypomagnesemia, also perhaps as a consquence of a magnesium loss from tissue. Infectious fever appears to be associated with a slight hypermagnesemia, while hypomagnesemia has been associated with acute infectious disease. Hypomagnesemia has also been found to be associated with the stress of surgery and in cases of myocardial infarction.

In general, the hypermagnesemia and hypomagnesemia observed after acute stresses do not appear to exert profound effects on normal physiological processes. But chronic stress that results in prolonged changes in serum magnesium, particularly hypomagnesemia, may lead to detrimental effects on the various systems of the body, particularly the cardiovascular system. The mechanisms involving the stress-induced changes in magnesium are not well understood.

SODIUM

Sodium is the principal cation in the extracellular fluids of the body, and its main fuction is to maintain osmotic equilibrium and proper volume of cells and body fluids. It plays a role in body acid-base balance. Sodium, along with potassium, participates in the elicitation of cell membrane electrical potentials. The underlying mechanisms involved in nerve conduction and muscular contraction require appropriate changes in electrical membrane potentials to occur. Sodium and potassium are intimately involved in such changes, and therefore the processes of nerve conduction and muscle contraction depend on the presence of adequate amounts of these two ions. Sodium by itself prevents excessive water loss from tissues, and both sodium and potassium play an important role in regulating the distribution of fluids in the body and in normal water balance.

Deficiency Conditions

Because sodium is present in a wide variety of foodstuffs, its deficiency in the human diet is uncommon. It is found combined with chlorine as common table salt. Foods rich in sodium are of animal origin and include meat, poultry, fish, eggs, and milk. Many types of food-processing methods use the salts of sodium. Examples of such processed foods are bacon, crackers, and some breads. Most people probably take in much more sodium daily than they actually need. However, sodium deficiency may occur in hot climates, particularly when sweating has been perfuse. A deficiency may result after vomiting or after the stress of strenuous physical exercise, particularly in hot weather. Deficiency symptoms include weight loss, weakness, possible nervous disorders, and neuralgia.

POTASSIUM

While sodium is the major cation in extracellular fluids, potassium is the major cation found in the intracellular fluids. It plays a role, along with sodium, calcium, and magnesium, in the normal excitability of nerve and muscle tissue, especially cardiac muscle.

In interacting with other elements, potassium participates in many enzymatic reactions involving protein and carbohydrate metabolism.

Potassium plays an important role along with sodium in regulating body fluid balance and fluid volume. It is equally important in helping to maintain the acid-base balance in the body. It maintains the alkaline part of the pH equilibrium. The level of potassium in the body has been used to determine lean body mass.

Deficiency Conditions

Potassium deficiency normally does not occur because of a lack in the diet. Other conditions, whether pharmacological or physiological, may precipitate a potassium deficiency. A high salt intake results in not only a sodium but also a potassium loss by the body. The repeated use of diuretic drugs results in a potassium loss as does persistent use of anticonstipation medications. Diarrhea, vomiting, fasting, starvation, and hypoglycemia can also precipitate a potassium loss.

Deficiency symptoms include weight loss, disorders of the nervous and muscular systems, irregular heart activity, and gastrointestinal disorders.

Sodium, Potassium, and Stress

The effects of stress on sodium and potassium levels in the blood are regulated by the circulating levels of the hormone aldosterone, the most important of a group of hormones (mineralocorticoids) secreted by the adrenal cortex. Aldosterone has a direct effect on the sodium concentration in the blood: it enhances the reabsorption of sodium by the renal tubules and therefore increases the level of sodium in the circulation. It is one of the important regulators of sodium concentration in the extracellular fluid compartment of the body. As aldosterone secretion increases, sodium reabsorption increases and circulating blood levels of sodium rise. On the other hand, the hormone has a reciprocal effect on potassium. Aldosterone enhances potassium secretion by the renal tubules, which in turn results in a potassium loss from the body. Increased levels of aldosterone in the circulation therefore result in a higher loss of potassium from the body. Under normal conditions, the secretion level of aldosterone maintains a proper body balance of the two electrolytes.

The secretion of aldosterone is influenced by the renin-angiotensin hormone system and the prevailing blood concentration of sodium. During the elicitation of the stress response, angiotensin II is increased in the circulation, and its increase appears to enhance the secretion of aldosterone. Elevated levels of aldosterone, as may occur during or as a result of the elicitation of the stress response, may ultimately result in increased levels of sodium in the blood, concomitant with some potassium loss.

Wohler (1972) describes the effects on serum sodium levels as a result of shipping stress in feeder cattle. Wohler demonstrates serum sodium levels to be elevated at the point of origin and at the point of destination, as well as one week after arrival for all groups of cattle studied. A stress-induced increase in aldosterone secretion may be implicated here. The hypersecretion of aldosterone, which occurs presumably as a result of the stress response, enhances renal sodium reabsorption, which in turn increases sodium levels in the blood. In this type of stress exposure, the increase in sodium retention of the cattle was maintained for 45 days after shipping, after which sodium levels returned to normal.

Paré and McCarthy (1966) describe a study that does not demonstrate a stress-induced increase in aldosterone. They subjected laboratory rats to a condition of chronic environmental stress. Although these animals did demonstrate a pronounced stress response, Paré and McCarthy did not observe a significant change in the sodium potassium electrolyte balance of the animals. They conclude from their study that while the exposure to chronic environmental stress does initiate a distinct activation of the pituitary adrenal glucocorticoid response, the adrenal mineralocorticoid (aldosterone) levels were not significantly affected and therefore the sodium potassium electrolyte balance was not markedly disturbed in these animals.

John and George (1977) report serum sodium to be increased and serum potassium to be decreased in pigeons as a result of heat stress. Steyn (1975) studied the effect of captivity stress in the baboon and reports elevated serum sodium and decreased serum potassium levels. On the other hand, Coburn et al. (1966) demonstrate enhanced aldosterone secretion and sodium retention during environmental heat stress exposure in humans. With regard to stress-induced changes in serum potassium levels in the body, they also describe certain characteristics of adaptation to heat stress. They state that the body's initial adaptation to heat stress results in a sodium retention and potassium loss (kaluresis), probably due to an increase in the secretion of aldosterone. During the course of the heat exposure, potassium may be lost as a result of decreased dietary intake and/or sweating. Therefore, under acute heat stress, potassium depletion may occur.

These studies suggest that more than one mechanism may be involved in the stress-induced changes in sodium retention in the body. The adrenal pituitary cortical (glucocorticoid) secretion with or without aldosterone production and/or activation of the sympathetic nervous system have all been implicated as factors that may be involved in the stress-induced enhancement of sodium in the body.

Other studies also demonstrate stress-induced changes in body sodium and potassium. Excretory electrolyte patterns in response to stress in reptiles is described by Spigel and Ramsay (1969). These researchers studied urinary sodium and potassium in electrically shocked turtles as compared to unshocked controls. Sodium and potassium excretion was significantly elevated as a result of shock and remained elevated for several days. The cation excretion patterns returned to normal only after the animals were placed in a new environment. These researchers suggest that the observed urinary electrolyte patterns may reflect the stress-induced activation of the renin-angiotensin system and aldosterone. The stress-induced increase in blood pressure mediated by increased levels of angiotensin may lead to decreases in the glomerular filtration rate, which in turn reduces sodium reabsorption. The reduced reabsorption of the cation will then result in a higher urinary excretion of sodium, as observed.

Other researchers report an increase in sodium retention and a potassium loss as a result of emotional stress (Moore 1953; Thorn et al. 1953; Tigranian et al. 1980) and an increase in sodium retention as a result of psychological stress (Grignolo et al. 1982; Light et al. 1983). Light et al. subjected young men to the stress of competitive mental tasks and found that the urinary sodium and fluid excretion was markedly reduced. These researchers found that the degree of sodium retention was directly associated in magnitude with the increase in heart rate during stress. These young men were chosen from a group who had either one or two hypertensive parents or who were borderline hypertensive. Tigranian et al. (1980) describe a study in which the sodium and potassium blood levels were measured in fifteen male students before and immediately after a state examination in medical school. They found that before the examination, the blood levels of aldosterone, sodium, and potassium were in the normal range. After the examination, aldosterone secretion increased but still remained within the normal range. However, these researchers found sodium levels to decrease (hyponatremia) after the examination, which could not have resulted from the increase in aldosterone levels. In addition, they found no change in potassium plasma levels both before and after the examination. Other researchers report a significant increase in blood aldosterone levels as a result of emotional stress in animals (Markoff et al. 1978; Clamage et al. 1976).

For many years it has been known that dietary salt intake could exert an influence on blood pressure. Today it is an accepted fact that there is a natriuretic (sodium) effect of blood pressure. A state of sodium retention is known to contribute to elevations in blood pressure. It is also known that several types of chronic stress are associated with elevations in blood pressure. The interrelationships among these variables, which may include other, unknown, factors, remain to be elucidated.

Potassium may also play an important role in the regulation of blood pressure. Potassium is closely linked to sodium regulation; it may exert its effect on blood pressure through sodium. Both sodium and potassium are actively transported across the cell membranes via a pump that is dependent upon the enzyme Na-K-ATPase. Changes in intracellular sodium or extracellular potassium stimulate Na-K-ATPase activity, and electrolyte transport across the cell membrane is increased, perhaps contributing to blood pressure changes. Potassium may act independently since both acute and chronic increases in extracellular potassium concentrations lower blood pressure (possibly mediated through an increase in Na-K-ATPase activity; Dyckner and Wester 1983). Magnesium must be present for Na-K-ATPase to properly function. Hence, at the cellular level, potassium may be exerting some influence on blood pressure regulation. Therefore, changes in plasma concentration and total body content of electrolytes, particularly sodium and potassium, can exert an influence not only in normal experimental subjects but also in both normotensive and hypertensive subjects (Louis and Spector 1975; Meneely and Battarbee 1976).

Raab et al. (1968) describe a study of the effect of isolation stress on myocardial electrolytes in rats. They report that prolonged isolation stress in laboratory rats was associated with a significant increase in myocardial sodium and a significant decrease in myocardial potassium, resulting in a decrease in the K-Na ratio. These electrolyte changes tended to be restored to baseline levels within a short time after the animals were returned to community life. In addition, epinephrine infusion induced a state of myocardial necrosis. Hemorrhages were also observed, which, as these researchers indicate, is attributed to the stress-induced adrenal glucocorticoid overactivity. The change in the K-Na ratio, reflecting prolonged sodium-accumulating and potassium-depleting states, is also consistent with adrenal cortical aldosterone overactivity.

In summary, the stress-induced changes in the body content of sodium and potassium generally result in increased levels of sodium, that is, a sodium retention (hypernatremia) and decreased levels of potassium or a potassium loss (kaluresis). The factors involved in these stress-induced changes appear to be aldosterone and the renin-angiotensin system. Several research findings also suggest the involvement of the sympathetic nervous system in the stress-induced changes in sodium retention, which could be important in the long-term regulation of blood pressure or hypertension. The relationships between the various hormones mentioned and between potassium, sodium, blood pressure elevation, the sympathetic nervous system and chronic stress exposure remain to be clarified.

CHLORINE

Chlorine, in the form of chloride, is an important anion (negative ion) found both in the intracellular and extracellular fluids. It is found within cells combined with sodium as sodium chloride or salt. It plays a role in electrolyte balance and functions along with sodium as a regulator of osmotic balance and acid-base balance. In addition, chloride aids in the digestive process in the stomach, since it is essential for the synthesis of hydrochloric acid. It is found in high concentration in gastric juice. Chloride also stimulates liver function. It helps to eliminate toxic waste material from the body, just as chlorine is sometimes used commercially in the process of water purification because of its detoxifying properties.

Deficiency Conditions

Chloride deficiency in the diet under normal conditions is not a major concern. However, chloride may be depleted from the body in the same manner as sodium. Loss of chloride can result from such conditions as diarrhea, vomiting, or excessive sweating.

Chloride deficiency is found in disease states such as the early stages of pneumonia, gastritis, malignancies, diabetes, and in fevers. Increased chlorides may be found in the body in such states as anemia and cardiac disease. However, under normal conditions, excess amounts of chloride in the body are excreted.

Chlorine and Stress

Little research connecting any direct changes in body chloride and various types of stress exposure is available. However, since chloride is found mainly combined with sodium in the body, any changes in body sodium levels mediated by chronic stress exposure will most likely result in parallel changes in chloride.

SILICON

Silicon, while necessary for some animals, has not been established as being essential for humans. However, some evidence indicates that it may be an important ingredient in the connective tissue between joints and organs in humans and a necessary part of the bone structure in animals.

Silicon is a common food additive and so its deficiency is highly unlikely. However, when present in excess amounts, as in mines, it can result in a disease called silicosis, which can be fatal.

Deficiency Conditions

No deficiency condition is known to humans but defects in bone development are known to occur in chicks.

Silicon and Stress

Not much is known about the relationship, if any, of silicon levels in the body and the experience of acute or chronic stress.

SULFUR

The mineral element sulfur is found in every living cell since all cells contain protein and all proteins contain some sulfur. Proteins are composed of amino acids and the source of sulfur comes from the amino acids cystine, cysteine, and methionine. Sulfur appears to be essential for the synthesis of collagen and keratin. It also forms an important ingredient of other substances used by the body, such as the B vitamins thiamine (B_1) and biotin, the hormone insulin, and the anticoagulant heparin, found in several body tissues. It helps the liver in the secretion of bile as it is an ingredient of taurine, an important constituent of bile acid. Sulfur is important for cellular oxidation and cellular energy production It plays a role in maintaining ion balance in tissues when oxidized to sulfate. This is very necessary for normal brain function. It plays a role in purifying the intestinal environment by combining with certain toxic or unwanted substances in the body, which eventually results in their elimination.

While present in every cell, sulfur is heavily concentrated in the skin, hair, and nails. It has been widely used topically in ointments to treat skin disorders such as dermatitis and psoriasis. It is also used as a skin toner. In this capacity it may be linked to selenium and zinc in maintaining healthy skin, hair, and nails. If the diet contains adequate amounts of protein, then most likely the sulfur requirements of the body are satisfied.

Deficiency Conditions

Symptoms of sulfur deficiency include skin disorders such as dermatitis and possibly eczema and psoriasis. Other symptoms include the imperfect development of hair and nails. Also, should there by any deficiency in the intake of protein, which contains the sulfur-containing amino acids, growth retardation may occur.

Sulfur and Stress

Not very much is known about the effects of various types of stress exposure and changes in body and tissue levels of sulfur. Because of the role sulfur plays in tissue respiration and carbohydrate metabolism (via insulin), the body probably needs more during the experience of stress.

6

THE TRACE MINERAL ELEMENTS

As described earlier, the body is also composed of mineral elements that are present in trace amounts (less than 0.01 percent). Some of these elements are known to have important physiological functions and some have been reported to be influenced by various types of stress.

ALUMINUM

Not much is known about the physiological role of aluminum in the human body or the role that it plays in human nutrition. However, it is found in many types of plants and animal foods. This element, when present in excess amounts, can have toxic effects. For this reason aluminum is discussed more generally in the chapter on toxic mineral elements (Chapter 7).

Aluminum and Stress

Not much is known about the effects of stress on the levels of aluminum in the body. However, its serum concentration has been shown to increase as a result of the stress of pulmonary infection while other disease states may exhibit depressed levels of this trace element.

ARSENIC AND CADMIUM

The requirements of these two minerals in humans has yet to be established, although arsenic is considered to be essential for growth in animals (Schwartz 1977). The physiological role of cadmium is only beginning to be recognized.

Deficiency Conditions

Deficiencies of both these trace elements have been shown to produce growth depression as well as malfunction of specific organs in certain animals.

Both arsenic and cadmium, when present in excess amounts in the body, have been shown to produce toxic effects. The presence of zinc may ameliorate the toxic effects of cadmium. For a further description of these trace mineral elements and their toxic effects, see Chapter 7.

CHROMIUM

Chromium is a trace mineral that plays a physiological role in both humans and animals and whose deficiency results in diabetes-like symptomatology. This mineral is associated with a glucose tolerance factor. Its precise relation to diabetes has yet to be determined but it appears to work in conjunction with insulin in carbohydrate metabolism, in maintaining normal blood sugar levels, and in the transport of glucose across cell membranes. It also functions in fat metabolism. Chromium may be involved in protein synthesis, since it is found within cells in association with nucleic acids.

Deficiency Conditions

A chromium deficiency may be prevalent in different populations throughout the United States. Its deficiency, as mentioned, results in abnormal levels of sugar in the blood. However, when insulin is secreted by the pancreas, the chromium, apparently being released from tissues, increases in the bloodstream. Chromium probably acts as a cofactor for insulin. It is considered to be necessary for insulin activity at a cellular level (Mertz et al. 1961), and therefore it is considered to play a role in glucose metabolism. In view of its role with insulin, chromium may be involved in the etiology of late-onset diabetes. If it is, that will certainly influence the future of clinical research in the area (Hsu 1979). Not only has it been observed that chromium levels decrease in diabetics but also that chromium levels decrease with age. For example, Canfield and Dorsy (1976) present a study in humans that demonstrates that total chromium concentration decreases with advancing years. Elderly subjects have been shown to have lower concentrations of chromium in their urine.

In animal experiments, a chromium deficiency results in abnormally high blood cholesterol levels and an increase in fat deposits in cardiac blood vessels. Also, a comparison of body chromium levels of people living in the West and the East shows that body levels of chromium are much lower in the West. Western people are much more prone to suffer from heart disease than those in the eastern part of the world. Hence, chromium deficiency may be linked to heart disease. Chromium is a suspected factor in arteriosclerosis, heart disease, and diabetes.

Chromium and Stress

Few studies describe chromium in relation to the stress response.

Mertz and Roginski (1969) report retarded growth and diminished longevity as a consequence of chromium deficiency in laboratory rats and mice raised in controlled environmental conditions. They found that rats subjected to the nutritional stress of a low-protein diet (10 percent) and chromium (<100 ppb) had a moderate growth supression, which dietary chromium supplementation alleviated. Subjecting the animals to the physical stress of controlled exercise or hemorrhage led to even more severe symptoms of the deficient chromium state. With the increasing severity of the applied stress, as after hemorrhage, there were greater differences between the chromium-deficient and chromium-supplemental group. Under the extreme conditions of experimental hemorrhage, chromium becomes an element essential for life.

This study points to the necessity of studying the role of chromium in the other conditions of human nutritional stress. One condition certainly worth investigating is the stress of protein malnutrition.

COBALT

Cobalt is an important mineral because it forms a necessary part of vitamin B_{12} (cobalamin) and therefore is necessary for the production of red blood cells. It also functions in growth, metabolism, and in maintaining a healthy nervous system.

While not much is known about the normal function of cobalt in the body, it is known that cobalt activates several enzyme systems *in vitro*.

Cobalt is found in a variety of foodstuffs, so it is readily available in the human dietary repertoire.

Deficiency Conditions

Deficiency symptoms of cobalt alone are not known. The only deficiency symptom recognized with regard to cobalt is that associated with a lack of vitamin B_{12}—anemia accompanied by the symptoms of listlessness and weakness.

Toxicity

Toxicity of cobalt can result in anorexia and a decrease in muscle coordination. The cardiomyopathy observd in some beer drinkers may be associated with the increased levels of cobalt.

Cobalt and Stress

Very little is known about the effect of various types of acute stress exposures on cobalt metabolism. Serum and tissue cobalt levels have been observed to be altered as a result of cell or tissue damage. In some cases increased levels in serum and tissue cobalt have been reported to increase, while in other cases serum and tissue levels of this trace metal have been reported to decrease as a result of various types of acute and chronic stress. The mechanisms involved in the stress-induced changes in body levels of cobalt are not very well known.

COPPER

Copper is an essential mineral element found in the adult human body in small amounts, generally in the range of about 80 to 100 milligrams. It is usually found associated with proteins. Copper is found in the liver at all times. It is also found in the brain, heart, and kidney tissue. If forms a part of several enzyme systems, plays a role in tissue respiration, bone growth, and in the formation of the skin pigment melanin. Copper plays a role in the storage and release of iron to form red blood cell hemoglobin and is therefore essential for the synthesis of hemoglobin. It is essential for the synthesis of phospholipids and for the production of ribonucleic acid (RNA). Copper plays a role in the utilization of vitamin C by the body. The concentration of copper appears to be highest at birth and during growth, and it appears to play a role in bone formation and maintenance of bone tissue.

Deficiency Conditions

Copper deficiency does not appear to be common in the United States. Copper deficiency symptoms include weakness, anemia (despite the presence of adequate amounts of iron), growth depression, skeletal defects, interference in iron metabolism, defects in pigmentation, changes in hair color, heart disease, and brain damage.

The use of oral contraceptive agents may result in elevated levels of serum copper. On the other hand, pregnancy may require a greater demand for copper as it is used by the fetus as well as the mother.

Copper and Stress

There is some evidence that the levels of serum copper are affected by various types of stress exposure. It has been reported that several disease states are associated with elevations in serum copper levels. Although this association could very well be the result of a general stress reaction, further investigative work is necessary to clarify this. Some chronic diseases characterized by increased serum copper concentrations are hypertension, diabetes mellitus, coronary atherosclerosis, and various blood disorders (Herring et al. 1960).

Brunia and Buyze (1972) report higher serum levels of copper (hypercupremia) in epileptic patients than healthy control individuals who were matched for both age and sex. These researchers determined serum copper levels of 94 epileptic children and 80 adult patients. They found that the serum copper levels of the different groups of patients were significantly higher than controls. Also, they report elevated serum copper levels for all types of epilepsy studied. In contrast, low serum copper levels have shown to be associated with ischemic heart disease. Heart disease is the leading cause of death in the United States, despite a recent decline. It is characterized by several factors, among which are glucose intolerance, abnormal electrocardiogram, hypercholesterolemia, and hyperuricemia. Similar characteristics have been found in copper-deficient animals (Klevay 1983). In humans with copper depletion, glucose intolerance and hypercholesteremia have also been observed (Klevay 1983).

A sex difference exists as far as serum copper levels are concerned. Copper concentrations appear to be much higher in females than males (Lahey et al. 1953). Also, the stress of pregnancy is characterized by an elevation in plasma copper levels.

Flynn et al. (1971a) found little or no correlation between the stress-induced increase in anterior pituitary secretion of ACTH and serum copper levels.

Some data indicate that elevated serum copper levels may be carcinogenic in humans. However, there is sparce epidemiological evidence to suggest any involvement of copper dietary sources and human carcinogensis.

In summary, the stress of some diseases appears to affect copper metabolism and result in hypercupremia. Examples are acute and chronic infections, myocardial infarction, leukemias, and various anemias and malignancies. Stress-induced hypercupremia is a function of the intensity and duration of the imposed stress. The mechanism underlying the stress-induced increase in copper metabolism is not well known and needs further clarification. For a more comprehensive review of the physiological role of copper in the body and its status in human nutrition, see Hsu (1979).

GALLIUM

Not very much is known about the physiological role of this trace element in the human body. However, it has been reported that blood gallium levels appear to be elevated in patients experiencing the stress of liver disease.

IODINE

Iodine forms an essential part of the hormones thyroxine and triiodothyronine, secreted by the thyroid gland. These hormones play a role in regulating the metabolic rate of the body. Because of this iodine is important among the trace minerals.

Most of the iodine in the body is concentrated in the thyroid gland although smaller amounts are present in other tissues, such as the gastric mucosa and salivary glands. Iodine is present in the mammary glands during the process of lactation. This trace element participates in several enzyme systems that are involved in growth, reproduction, lactation, and energy release.

Deficiency Conditions

Iodine deficiency results in a condition known as goiter and is characterized by an enlarged thyroid gland and hypothyroidism. The deficiency is generally dietary in origin since this condition appears to be associated with specific geographical regions of the world. However, other factors such as infectious agents or defects in the enzyme system responsible for thyroid hormone production should not be ruled out.

The deficiency symptoms include physical and mental sluggishness. Should a deficiency of this trace mineral occur before puberty, possible depression in physical and mental development leading to cretinism can result.

Limited data suggest an involvement of iodine deficiency and the risk of thyroid cancer in humans. However, evidence to date is not conclusive.

Iodine and Stress

Certain conditions of stress appear to interfere with proper thyroid functioning. The stress of pregnancy and the stress of adolescent growth, particularly in girls, requires a greater demand for thyroid hormones and therefore iodine. Women are susceptible to iodine deficiency during menopause. Also, a continual exposure to cold requires a greater amount of iodine in the diet than under normal conditions.

IRON

Iron is a mineral element absolutely necessary for life and is found in every living cell, acting as a stimulant for many cellular processes. The normal adult human contains about 3 to 5 grams of iron. It is an essential component of certain respiratory enzymes, particularly the cytochrome system. Iron also participates in several enzyme systems involved in energy production via the metabolism of proteins, carbohydrates, and fats.

It is present in the liver, spleen, and bone marrow and is required by the bone marrow in the synthesis of red blood cells. The highest percentage of iron is found in red blood cells as a constituent of hemoglobin. Hemoglobin is a complex molecule that acts as a carrier for oxygen and carbon dioxide. It carries oxygen from the lungs and releases it to the tissues and picks up carbon dioxide from the tissues and transports it to the lungs. Iron is also found in muscle cells as a constituent of myoglobin. Myoglobin, in contrast to hemoglobin, is used to store the oxygen necessary for muscle contraction. Iron is also present in the body and stored in tissues in smaller amounts bound to protein. This form of iron is referred to as ferritin or hemosiderin. Iron may also be involved in the structure of polyribosomes and may therefore play a role in protein synthesis.

Iron is essential for the proper utilization of the B vitamins by the body. For the effective assimilation of iron by the body, vitamin C and copper, cobalt, and manganese are necessary. The only way the body can lose a significant amount of iron is through a loss of blood. Under normal conditions, little iron is lost from the body. Most of the iron released from cells and tissues is recycled by the body and reused.

Deficiency Conditions

Iron deficiency is common in the United States as well as in other countries and mainly comes from dietary factors. The most common iron deficiency disorder is anemia. (A deficiency of vitamin B_{12} and folacin also results in anemia.) Other deficiency symptoms are a decreased amount of red blood cells, a decreased amount of hemoglobin, a pale complexion, weakness, fatigue, loss of vitality, and susceptibility to infections. Some evidence indicates that iron deficiency may result in a depression of the immune response (Chandra 1975; Chandra et al. 1977; MacDougall et al. 1975).

Women are very prone to develop iron deficiency (as well as calcium deficiency). Much iron can be lost through menstruation and blood loss at childbirth. Even though women absorb iron more efficiently than men, they may experience iron deficiency because of a low dietary intake of the mineral through their choice of foods. Hence, in many cases iron supplementation is recommended. Frequent blood loss from hemorrhoids, ulcers, or any illness where blood is lost and prolonged use of aspirin can also predispose one to a condition of iron deficiency. Pregnant women and growing children are likely to experience an iron-deficiency anemia because of their added need for iron.

Since many oral contraceptives reduce blood loss during menstruation, iron deficiency may not occur when these drugs are used. However, during pregnancy and lactation, the mother loses iron to the infant, and her iron requirements necessarily increase.

Persistent use of highly processed foods deficient in copper will lower the iron content of the body and result in a deficiency. Diets that do not contain enough iron-containing foods may result in a lack of adequate amounts of iron in the body.

Consumption of large amounts of coffee or tea may exert an inhibiting effect on iron absorption in the body.

Iron deficiency has also been implicated in cancers of the gastrointestinal tract, including the stomach and esophagus, although to date, the data are not conclusive.

Iron, Other Associated Plasmatic Factors, and Stress

Balasch and Flos (1975) studied several factors related to iron and copper metabolism in rats exposed to immobilization stress. They found that after one hour of immobilization, both the ferroxidase activity and plasmatic copper decreased. They further found that after 6 hours, the plasmatic iron levels were lower, while at 15 hours the values returned to normal. This work suggests a possible link between changes in iron, copper, and ACTH release during stress. A possible role for increased levels of zinc is mentioned. Other researchers have found immobilization stress to influence several plasmatic factors, including iron, copper, total ferroxidase activity, and zinc (Bonfils et al. 1958). Flos and Armario (1978) studied the effect of adrenaline administration on iron, copper, and zinc levels in plasma and spleen and copper, zinc, and manganese levels in liver. Other tissues were also studied. They found no significant short-term effect of adrenaline admininstration. However, other researchers demonstrate that ACTH significantly influences the iron, copper, and zinc levels in the liver and iron levels in the spleen immediately after subcutaneous ACTH injection (Armario et al. 1978).

Animal studies that demonstrate a fall in serum iron levels as a result of the stress of infection are described by Weinberg (1974, 1978) and Kluger and Rothenburg (1979).

Some research reports involving human subjects demonstrate that serum iron concentration rapidly decreases as a result of various types of stress exposure. Feldthusen et al. (1953) first described the change in serum iron levels as a result of operative stress. They report a decrease in serum iron levels (hypoferremia) postoperatively and suggest that this hypoferremia may be the result of the activation of the stress mechanism in the body. Syrkis and Machtey (1973) and Fitzsimons and Kaplan (1980) studied patients with acute myocardial infarction and observed a rapid fall in serum iron concentration. They suggest that this decrease may be the result of the stress associated with such a condition. Ballantyne (1983) reports a rapid drop in serum iron levels after elective cholecystectomy. This researcher reports that serum iron concentration rapidly decreases from preoperative levels to postoperative levels in 50 patients undergoing elective cholecystectomy. Ballantyne reports that after surgery, the serum iron levels slowly return to normal. In addition, Ballantyne suggests that the postoperative low serum levels of iron may be a purposeful metabolic response to the stress of surgery, a stress-induced nonspecific metabolic response that serves to protect the organism against infection.

Weinberg (1974) has observed low serum iron levels in several patients experiencing various types of infections. In addition, Fitzsimons and Levine (1983) observed a rapid drop in serum iron concentration in four categories of patients subjected to surgical, infectious, neurological, and obstetric stressful events. They suggest that the observed phenomenon of hypoferremia in all cases studied appears to be a nonspecific response to these stressful situations.

In summary, several types of stress exposure, both acute and chronic, have been shown to depress serum iron concentrations. Such stress includes infectious illnesses, various malignancies, surgery, trauma, and malnutrition. The transient hypoferremia observed after acute stress may not result in any major clinical consequences but may play some as yet unknown role in resisting the effects of stress. Further investigative work needs to be done to explain the underlying mechanisms involved in the observed rapid fall or iron and other associated plasmatic factors as a result of various types of stress exposures.

MANGANESE

This essential trace mineral is necessary for growth, thyroxine synthesis, reproduction, proper functioning of the gastrointestinal system, and the healthy functioning of the nervous system. It plays a role in the synthesis of nucleic acids and it participates in enzyme systems involved in cholesterol synthesis and in fat metabolism. It serves as a cofactor in the reactions involving oxidative phosphorylation. Manganese also aids in the activation of enzymes necessary for the body's use of vitamin B_1, biotin, choline, and vitamin C.

Deficiency Conditions

No clear deficiency states of manganese are known to exist. Possible manganese deficiency symptoms are retardation in growth, depressed tissue respiration, ataxia, abnormal estrus cycles, and offspring with skeletal and pancreatic defects.

Toxicity

Toxic doses of manganese may occur in industrial workers who breathe in large amounts of the metal. Mental disturbances and disorders of the muscular system may be a result of toxic levels of the metal in the body.

Manganese and Stress

Manganese is a trace element that is used widely in industry, particularly in several types of fuel systems. It is known that industrial workers exposed to more than normal amounts of manganese can develop a neurological disorder (Chandra et al. 1974; 1979).

Chandra et al. (1979) describe the effect of immobilization stress exposure on the response of rat brain to manganese. They report that chronic immobilization stress did not alter the manganese balance of the central nervous system. In addition, after immobilization stress exposure was combined with manganese salt injections, a modification of the brain tissue content of norepinephrine, dopamine, tyrosine, and tryptophan occurred. The significance of this change in brain amino acids and amines needs to be further clarified. According to their findings, Chandra et al. (1979) suggest that the neurotoxic effects of manganese may be enhanced as a result of exposure to physical stress. Other researchers have also found changes in brain amino acids in brain tissue as a result of stress exposure (Curzon et al. 1972; and Curzon and Green, 1969). The implication of this research as applied to the human situation suggests that increased exposure to manganese as well as to physical stress may enhance the neurotoxic effects of the metal on the human central nervous system. Further investigative work needs to be done to clarify such relationships.

Not very much work has been reported on the stress-induced changes in manganese metabolism. The stress of acute radiation influences oxidative phosphorylation and mitochondrial energy production, all of which are known to involve the activity of manganese. Also, not too much research is available to indicate that a variety of stresses significantly alter manganese metabolism or serum and tissue manganese levels.

MOLYBDENUM

Molybdenum is an important trace element present in many enzyme systems of the body. It participates in the metabolism of carbohydrates and fats. It is an essential part of an enzyme system (the xanthine oxidase system) responsible for iron metabolism and for the conversion of certain protein substances into uric acid. Excessive levels of molybdenum may lead to high uric acid production, with a subsequent condition of gout.

Deficiency Conditions

No deficiency condition for molybdenum is known. However, there is evidence that high levels of copper in the diet are antagonistic to molybdenum and may be a cause for concern.

Molybdenum and Stress

Not very much is known about the effects of stress and molybdenum levels in body tissues. However, in view of its role in carbohydrate and fat metabolism, intense or chronic stress may increase the body's need for this trace element. Further research is necessary to clarify any relationship that may exist between the experience of stress and molybdenum levels in the body.

NICKEL

Nickel has recently been discovered in human tissue in large amounts. Its function in the body is not known. Therefore, it has not been established as a necessary trace element for humans. Nickel plays a role in the hydrogenation of vegetable oils. Perhaps this may provide an insight into its physiological role in the body. However, it has been shown that nickel is necessary for chicks, rats, and pigs.

Deficiency Conditions

No deficiency conditions of nickel are known to exist in humans. Nickel deficiency in animals has resulted in retarded growth of the young and possible liver damage.

Nickel and Stress

Some researchers report that serum nickel levels increase rapidly after the stress of acute myocardial infarction (Sunderman et al. 1970). Some research describes an inhibitory activity of nickel on the anterior pituitary secretion of prolactin *in vivo* and *in vitro* (Labella et al. 1973a, 1973b; and Carlson 1984). Nickel has also been reported to be inhibitory to stimulated growth hormone secretion (Dormer et al. 1973). It is known that both these hormones are increased in secretion as a result of the stress response. The means by which nickel exerts its inhibitory effect is not entirely clear, although some researchers suggest that nickel may act as a calcium antagonist in the mechanism of stimulus-secretion coupling (Carlson 1974; Dormer et al. 1973). Further research is needed to explore whether nickel may play a role in other hormonal secretory mechanisms of the body under both stressed and nonstressed conditions.

SELENIUM

Selenium belongs to the same chemical group of elements as sulfur. It is found in soil and grains and has several commercial uses, such as in rectifiers, photocells, and dandruff shampoo.

Selenium is considered to be an essential nutrient for both humans and animals.

Selenium appears to act in concert with vitamin E. Both are antioxidants, that is, they prevent any destructive effects of oxidation on cells, such as a slowing down of chemical reactions as a result of aging. This mineral may help in preventing hardening of tissues due to oxidation and therefore plays a role in maintaining a youthful tone and elasticity of body tissues. Selenium aids in reproduction, being one of the constituents of semen in males. Half of the selenium in the body of a male is found in the seminal glands and testicles, adjacent to the prostate gland.

Selenium may also play a protective role against certain types of heart disease, angina, high blood pressure, and cancer. Much evidence indicates that selenium added to either the diet or the drinking water protects against tumor development induced by various chemical carcinogenic agents.

Deficiency Conditions

There is evidence that selenium may counteract the effects of heavy metals such as cadmium, which is often found in tobacco smoke. Smokers may therefore have a greater need for selenium. Selenium may offset the harmful effects of other heavy metals such as mercury (from pesticides, seaweed) and arsenic (from pollution). Hence, an increased exposure to these heavy metals may enhance the body's need for selenium. More investigative efforts are needed to substantiate any claims of a selenium deficiency in the presence of these toxic mineral elements.

Dandruff is one symptom that may have a possible link to selenium deficiency. In many instances, the use of a selenium-treated shampoo can control a dandruff condition.

Selenium and Stress

Not too much is known about the effects of stress on the levels of selenium in the body. However, some research describes the role of selenium and the stress of certain malignancies.

Many animal experiments show that selenium exerts a protective effect against certain types of cancer. Experiments have been performed on both viral and carcinogen-induced cancers, and both types have been shown to be prevented by selenium. Several epidemiological studies suggest an anticarcinogenic effect of selenium in humans showing serum selenium levels to be lower in certain cancer patients than in control subjects (Allaway et al. 1968; McConnell et al. 1980; Calautti et al. 1980; Willett et al. 1983). Some researchers, in exploring the mechanism of action of the anticarcinogenic effect of selenium, report that it enhances the primary immune response, or, in other words, acts as a stimulant to the immune system (Spallholz et al. 1975). Continued investigative work is necessary to clarify the role and mechanism of action of selenium as a cancer protective agent. For a review of this subject, see Helzlsouer (1983).

STRONTIUM

Not very much is known about the role strontium plays in the body and therefore this element has not yet been firmly established as necessary in human nutrition. However, it is known that strontium is a necessary trace mineral element found in bones.

Deficiency Conditions

To date, no deficiency conditions are known to exist for strontium in humans.

Strontium and Stress

Not very much is known about the effects of acute or chronic stress on the levels of strontium in the body.

TIN

The trace element tin has not yet been firmly established as necessary for humans although it has been accepted as necessary for rats.

Deficiency Conditions

To date, no deficiency conditions are known to exist for tin in humans. However, growth retardation occurs as a result of tin deficiency in several animal species.

Tin and Stress

Not very much is known about the effects of acute or chronic stress on the levels of tin in the body.

ZINC

Zinc is a trace element found in the human adult in amounts from 1.4 to 2.3 grams (average 1.8 grams) and is a necessary constituent of more than 100 enzyme systems of the body. It plays a role in several enzyme systems involved in metabolism and is an integral part of the enzyme system that is involved in red blood cell carbon dioxide transport from the tissues to the lungs. Therefore, zinc plays a role in maintaining the body's acid-base balance. Zinc performs several other roles in the body. It is necessary in the synthesis of DNA and proteins. The absorption of several of the vitamins, especially the B complex vitamins, require the presence of zinc. Zinc is important for normal brain function and for the development of the reproductive organs. Zinc is necessary for the synthesis of the male sex hormone, testosterone. It is found throughout most of the male reproductive system. It is present in high concentration in sperm and is therefore necessary for normal reproductive activity. It is found in high concentrations in the heart, pituitary gland, adrenal glands, kidney, and pancreas. It is involved in the storage and secretion of insulin. Since it is found in various endocrine glands, it may play a role in several hormonal secretions besides insulin. There is some indication that zinc supplementation results in a lowering of blood cholesterol. Patients with atherosclerosis exhibit some improvement after receiving zinc supplementation. Zinc also plays a role in accelerating the body's healing process. Some recent reports state that zinc may have an antiviral effect and may aid in the relief of the common cold. However, this is a subject for further investigative scientific work. For a more comprehensive treatment of the recent advances in zinc metabolism, see Prasad et al. (1982).

Deficiency Conditions

Slow healing of wounds is one of the characteristics of a zinc deficiency. A loss of the sense of taste and smell may also be related to a zinc deficiency. Sometimes such conditions may develop after a serious illness when the body's zinc levels have been found to be low. Zinc deficiency may result in growth retardation, hypogonadism, and decreased ACTH secretion. Lowered zinc levels have also been associated with a loss of appetite. Investigations are presently underway to study the effects of zinc intake on obesity. A deficiency in zinc can result in an inability of the intestinal walls to absorb food, which would result in a weakness and a lack of energy. A deficiency in zinc may also retard the growth process.

Zinc may play a role in immune responsiveness (Chandra 1980; Fracker et al. 1978; Fernandes et al. 1979; Gross et al. 1979). Chandra (1980) observed that the thymus gland of zinc-deficient animals weighed less than animals fed a zinc-controlled diet. A definite observed atrophy and hypofunction of the thymus gland was associated with a zinc deficiency in this study. The data presented are consistent with the fact that zinc deprivation results in a significant decrease in cell-mediated immune responses.

Conditions characterized by low body zinc levels include diabetes, excessive alcoholic intake, a diet heavy in processed foods, and the use of oral contraceptives and drugs.

Adding zinc to the diet appears to increase the need for vitamin A.

Toxicity

There is some indication that excessive amounts of zinc decrease immune responsiveness. High levels of body zinc appear to disrupt copper use and iron metabolism in the body. Large amounts of zinc appear to significantly decrease high-density lipoprotein concentrations and slightly increase low-density lipoprotein levels, thereby influencing cholesterol levels in the blood. Again, this subject requires further investigative effort.

Zinc and Stress

Several studies describe the effects of various types of stress exposure on plasma levels of zinc. Many of these studies demonstrate a decrease in the levels of plasma zinc in both humans and animals. Such stresses as acute infection (Pekarek et al. 1970; Vikbladh 1951; Corrigal et al. 1976), pregnancy (Hambidge and Droegemueller 1974) and postoperative shock and trauma (Lindeman et al. 1972; Hallbook and Hedelin 1977) have been reported. The changes occurring in plasma zinc levels as a result of stress have been attributed to an increase in its urinary excretion (Hallbook and Hedelin 1977) and to an increase in uptake of the metal, especially by the liver (Kincaid et al. 1976; Sugawara et al. 1983; Brady 1981). Another factor involved in the zinc loss associated with stress may have to do with increased protein catabolism and the increase in the amount of amino acids in the plasma (Henkin and Smith 1972).

Sandstead et al. (1966) describe the relationship between overt zinc deficiency and decreased levels of ACTH. ACTH, along with the glucocorticoids, increases as a result of stress of almost any type. ACTH has been shown to lower plasma zinc levels (Falchuk 1977) while the corticosteroids have been shown to enhance cellular uptake of zinc *in vitro* (Cox and Ruckenstern 1971). Flynn et al. (1971a) studied the condition of hypotensive stress exposure in laboratory rats. They studied ACTH and zinc levels during control, stress, and stress recovery periods. Throughout their study, they found parallel changes in ACTH and zinc, both increasing during stress and both decreasing during the stress recovery period.

In a subsequent work, Flynn et al. (1972) studied the *in vitro* effect of zinc in isolated adrenal glands on ACTH-induced stimulation of corticosterone synthesis. They observed a functional dependence of ACTH on serum zinc levels. If the *in vivo* situation (intact animal preparation) exhibits a functional dependence of ACTH on zinc, it follows that laboratory animals that are zinc deficient should exhibit signs of a decrease in corticosteroid production. To study this, Reeves et al. (1977) examined the effect of zinc-deficient laboratory rats on corticosterone synthesis, under stimulation by exogenous ACTH and two different stress conditions. They found that young zinc-deficient male rats respond with a normal release of corticosterone when exposed to stress or given exogenous ACTH, while zinc-deficient female rats subjected to the stress of pregnancy, surgery, and birth demonstrate a subnormal response.

In another study Flynn et al. (1971b) report that in seriously ill burn patients, massive doses of steroids have the effect of rapidly lowering levels of serum zinc. Their work further emphasizes the role of the anterior pituitary adrenal cortical axis in maintaining circulating zinc levels.

In contrast, Wegner et al. (1972) show that serum zinc was not significantly altered in dairy cattle given a corticotropin injection. They did not find any correlation between plasma corticosteroids and zinc levels. In addition, they demonstrate lowered zinc levels in animals subjected to hyperthermal and clinical ketosis stress. They observed that cows with mastitis (udder infection) had higher zinc levels than did controls. The effect of milking had no effect on serum zinc levels. The results of Wegner et al. seem in general to agree with those of Flynn et al. (1971b) and others, in that various stress exposures stimulate corticosteroid production and depress overall serum zinc levels. Further work is necessary to clarify the relationships involved in the activity of the pituitary adrenal cortical axis and serum zinc levels.

Another study investigating normal and zinc-deficient states is reported by Weisenberg et al. (1968). Pigs with normal levels of zinc, when subjected to the stress of infection, demonstrated lowered plasma zinc levels and survived. However, zinc-deficient pigs subject to the same stressor—infection—exhibited plasma-zinc concentrations that failed to fall more than their already low values. One third of these animals did not survive. On the other hand, Chesters and Will (1981) suggest that although a normal animal responds with lowered zinc levels when exposed to stress, zinc supplementation, in excess of normal dietary requirements, will not prove beneficial.

The physiological significance of the decrease in plasma levels of zinc as a consequence of stress is not entirely known. Perhaps these decreased zinc levels have some bearing on the necessary protection and survival of the organism in the face of stress. This is borne out by studies of the positive protective effect of zinc on gastric ulceration in laboratory animals induced by various types of stress exposure (Cho and Ogle 1977, 1978; Cho et al. 1980). Cho et al. (1980) demonstrate a possible mechanism involved in this protective effect of zinc. For a more comprehensive review of zinc and the effects of stress on serum zinc levels, see Hsu (1979), Chesters (1978), and Schloen et al. (1979).

In summary, a variety of stress exposures in both humans and animals have been shown to alter zinc metabolism and result in decreased levels of serum zinc. The stress associated with acute and chronic liver disease, infection, trauma, surgery, myocardial infarction, tumors, malignancies, leukemia, and anemia all result in depressed serum zinc levels. On the other hand, increased zinc levels associated with disease states or stress have generally not been observed.

The changes in zinc metabolism as a result of acute stress occur rapidly and perhaps may be useful in clinical diagnosis. However, the mechanisms involved in the stress-induced changes in zinc remain to be clarified. In some cases, the change may be of benefit to the organism, whereas in other cases, particularly under chronic conditions, a zinc deficit may prove harmful to the organism in the long term.

The type, chronicity, and intensity of the stressor, the degree of stress as perceived by the subject involved, and the participation of other physiological systems all have their bearing on the final results observed. All of these factors should be considered when reviewing the stress-induced changes in zinc or the relationships involved in the stress-induced changes in other body nutrients.

LITHIUM AND RUBIDIUM

For the sake of completeness, mention is made of these two mineral elements that, while not functioning in any known physiological role in the body, are used in the treatment of mental disorders.

Lithium is the lightest element and it is widely distributed in nature. It is present in the body in trace amounts. It is used in the treatment of mania and manic depression.

Rubidium is also not considered an essential trace element although it is present in minute amounts in the body. Its physiological role is unknown.

In the early part of the century, rubidium was used as an hypnotic and in the treatment of various nervous disorders. Today, it appears to be helpful in the treatment of depression. More research is needed to investigate its antidepressant properties and to clarify its role in the treatment of mental disorders.

Toxicity

Therapeutic blood levels of lithium are close to toxic levels. Therefore, when it is used in treatment, blood levels should be monitored closely and carefully. Toxic symptoms are drowsiness, diarrhea, and muscle weakness, among others. The use of lithium may also compromise sodium balance and thyroid function.

7

THE TOXIC MINERAL ELEMENTS

Several mineral elements are present in many processed food items, over-the-counter remedies, household items, and our natural environment, such as the air, lakes, rivers, and oceans. Excess amounts of these elements can be toxic. They upset normal physiological functioning and nutritional balance, primarily affecting the functioning of the brain and the nervous system. This is generally followed by other organ and system dysfunctioning. This sequence of events is similar to that observed in various nutritional deficiency states. The illnesses prominent in our society today that appear to parallel the increase in industrial technological development include the prevalence of mental diseases, learning disabilities, hyperactivity in children, respiratory disorders, heart disease, and cancer. In view of this, it is certainly worth investigating whether any correlation exists between the increase in the presence of these toxic mineral elements in our environment as a result of industrial technology and the prevalence of such disorders in society today. On the basis of the evidence now available, however, it appears plausible to adapt precautionary methods in which modern technological development can continue to grow and expand along with the curbing of the presence of toxic mineral elements in our immediate environment.

The main toxic mineral elements in question are aluminum, cadmium, fluorine, lead, mercury, and vanadium. Other, less toxic, elements are arsenic, beryllium, bismuth, and bromine.

ALUMINUM

Aluminum is a trace element, but if present in excess amounts in the body it can initiate toxic effects and can even be fatal. There is as yet no clearly established role of aluminum in human nutrition, but it is found in small amounts in many plant and animal foods. Aluminum is absorbed by the body and appears to be found in larger amounts in the brain, lungs, and liver. A main source of aluminum in the body is the use of aluminum foil and cookware. Minute quantities of the element may be absorbed into food during cooking. Another source of aluminum may be aluminum sulfate in drinking water. Aluminum sulfate is used in the process of water purification and may not be completely filtered out. Aluminum may also be found in some baking powders, white flour, antacids, aspirin tablets, toothpastes, deodorants, and as a base material in false teeth.

Some research describes an impairment of nerve and brain function in the presence of toxic doses of aluminum in laboratory animals. Other researchers report the induction of seizures (Kopeloff et al. 1942) and learning impairment (Crapper et al. 1973) in animals exposed to high doses of aluminum. Increased levels of aluminum have also been found in the brains of patients suffering from Alzheimer's disease and may account for some forms of dementia. Symptoms of gastrointestinal discomfort and inflammation have also been reported.

Deficiency Conditions

There are no clear deficiency symptoms of this heavy metal and no available information on its beneficial effects in human health and the prevention of disease.

ARSENIC

Arsenic is found in nature distributed throughout the waters and soils of many countries. Arsenic is also found in trace amounts in foods. Since it is used in insecticides, it may be present in some foods as a contaminant. While arsenic is generally considered to be a toxic element, individual susceptibility to arsenic toxicity is variable in the face of the many different chemical forms in which it is found. Therefore, the human dietary and toxic levels for arsenic have not yet been determined.

Arsenic has been found to be associated with cancer in humans but not in experimental laboratory animals. Perhaps under the conditions studied, humans may be more sensitive to the carcinogenic effects of arsenic than animals. At any rate, epidemiological evidence indicates that the risk of lung cancer in humans is increased as a result of the inhalation of arsenic compounds due to environmental contamination. Epidemiological evidence is also available linking arsenic contamination of drinking water with an increase in the risk of human skin cancer.

BERYLLIUM

This element is heavily used in industry, particularly in aircraft and rockets because of its extremely high heat-resistant properties. It is also used in several electronic devices, in the steel industry, in alloys, and in many common household items.

However, when the element is absorbed into the bloodstream, it is known to have several toxic effects in the body. Besides interfering with the function of such vital organs as the lungs and the heart, it interferes with the functioning of several important enzyme systems.

Breathing in beryllium dust can lead to serious respiratory disorders. It appears that this metal also has the ability to decrease the body's stores of magnesium, thus leading to further mineral imbalance and heart disease.

At present, there is no clear indication of an important physiological role of this substance in the body.

BISMUTH

Several compounds used in the relief of gastrointestional disturbances include the salts of bismuth. Prolonged use of such substances can result in toxic effects, causing disturbances of the nervous and muscular systems that may include such symptoms as mental confusion, possible impairment of memory, and muscle spasms.

At present, there is no clear indication of an important physiological role of this substance in the body.

BROMINE

This element is a halogen and belongs to the same class of chemical elements as fluorine, chlorine, and iodine. When absorbed in excessive amounts in the body, it can produce a series of toxic effects, including irritability, weakness, fatigue, mental sedation, and a depression of mental functioning. Thought processes may be slowed down, coupled with memory impairment.

Salts of bromine may be absorbed into the body as a result of the use of over-the-counter medications prescribed for the relief of gastrointestinal disturbances such as acid indigestion.

At present, there is no clear indication of the beneficial effects of bromine in human health and the prevention of disease.

CADMIUM

Cadmium only recently is beginning to be recognized as having some possible physiological function even though it has been considered a toxic substance for years.

Cadmium belongs to the same chemical group as mercury and zinc. In nature, it is found in close association with zinc, and its chemical activity is similar to that of zinc. Cadmium, because of its heat-resistant properties, is widely used in the enamel and plastics industry and in batteries (nickel-cadmium).

Cadmium in high enough doses is extremely toxic. The main sources of toxicity are some of the plant fungicides on the market. High levels of cadmium are also found in sewer sludge. Cadmium may be present in phosphate rock, and therefore its toxic effects would primarily affect the animal feed industry. Cadmium, along with mercury and selenium, has been labeled highly toxic by the Association of American Feed Control officials. Serum kidney and liver cadmium levels increase in clinical cases of bronchial carcinoma (Morgan 1970). In addition, environmental exposure to cadmium has been associated with an increase in the risk of kidney and prostate cancer. However, more evidence is needed to substantiate any role of cadmium exposure and carcinogensis in humans. Some of the toxic effects of cadmium are renal tubular necrosis, bone marrow hypoplasia, anemia, lymphocytopenia, ventricular hypertrophy, and hypertension.

FLUORINE

Fluorine is a member of the halogen family of chemical elements and is rarely found in the free state. It is found mostly in the combined state as fluoride.

Traces of fluorine, have been found in the skin, thyroid gland, bones, and teeth. It has been shown that fluoride (fluorine salt) enhances the density of bone in people suffering from osteoporosis and is important for dental health, particularly in growing children and adolescents. Hence, the basic importance of fluoride lies in its ability to lower the chances of dental caries and to strengthen bone structure. Fluoride is placed in the drinking water in many localities. The acceptable level is one part per million. In practically all localities where water fluoridation was introduced, dental caries in children has been lowered by 50 percent or greater. There are also indications that fluoride may aid in calcium retention in the bone structure of older people.

Fluorides are relatively safe when taken in small quantities but can have definite toxic effects when taken in higher doses. The toxic effect of fluorides occurs principally in the form of damage to both bones and teeth.

Contamination of the environment due to the presence of fluorides occurs mainly from industrial emissions, such as that associated with steel production, and phosphate and aluminum processing. Fluoride contamination may also come from the use of pesticides that contain fluorsilicates or fluoracetates.

Deficiency Conditions

Fluoride deficiency appears to result in tooth decay. No other deficiency symptoms are presently known.

LEAD

Lead, in trace amounts, has recently been shown to be necessary for growth and reproduction in rats. However, it has not been established as a necessary trace element in humans. It is known to be highly toxic. Lead poisoning can be a result of environmental pollution or chronic exposure to such substances as paints, grease, oils, old batteries, automobile exhausts, atmospheric dust, and deteriorating housing. The daily ingestion of only 1 milligram of lead can result in clinical toxicity. Lead may enter the body either through the gastrointestinal tract or through the skin. The main toxic effects of lead include damage to the central nervous system, brain dysfunction (encephalopathy), and damage to the gastrointestinal tract. Other toxic effects are seizure disorders, neuromuscular disturbances, anemia, possible blindness, and death.

Several researchers demonstrate that certain concentrations of lead significantly interfere with the process of learning in animals without affecting morbidity or mortality. In particular, Laporte and Talbott (1978), in a review of the subject, state that the presence of lead appears to have damaging effects on learning. They imply that even low concentrations of lead can have deleterious effects on higher levels of cognition. Human learning studies focus on the effects of various levels of lead in the body and the development of mental retardation and brain damage (Zarkowsky 1975; Beattie et al. 1975; National Research Council 1971). Hyperactivity in children has been associated with acute lead poisoning by some researchers. Many of the human research studies demonstrate varying results. This could be a result of a lack of proper or adequate controls (Laporte and Talbott 1978) or a lack of precisely defining the parameters under which the experimental conditions were carried out.

In animal research, it has been observed that high amounts of lead are tumorigenic in mice and rats. In humans, however, little epidemiological evidence indicates any association between dietary lead intake and the risk of cancer. Also, the exposure to high levels of lead in the environment has not been associated with an increased risk of cancer in humans.

Increased dietary levels of both calcium and phosphorus have been shown in some cases to override some of the effects of lead toxicity (Berg et al. 1980).

MERCURY

Mercury is the only metallic element that exists as a liquid at ordinary room temperatures. It has no known function in human nutrition. Arab physicians as far back as 600 B.C. used mercury for its medicinal properties (Sell 1974). Until recently, it was used clinically as a diuretic. In appropriate doses, mercury can be toxic to both humans and animals. Today, compounds of mercury are used commercially as pesticides and fungicides. Symptoms of toxicity in humans are kidney damage, vomiting, diarrhea, central nervous system damage, neurological damage, depression, growth suppression, and death.

In instances of human toxicity, the causes of mercury poisoning arise from contaminated meats and seeds that have been pretreated with mercurial fungicides.

VANADIUM

Vanadium is a trace element that has been shown to retard the formation of cholesterol in the vasculature of the body. Therefore it may help in the prevention of heart attacks. It has also been shown that vanadium in micro amounts enhances the rate of growth and increases the amount of hemoglobin in the bloodstream.

Vanadium is widely present in nature and is commonly found in phosphate sources. In higher doses it is found in fuel oil debris and can produce toxic effects in animals. Some of the toxic effects include growth retardation, dehydration, diarrhea, weakness, and death (National Research Council 1980).

Deficiency Conditions

No deficiency condition at present is known for vanadium. For a more comprehensive treatment of the stress induced by these toxic elements, see Richie (1984).

HAIR ANALYSIS

Hair analysis is a process that provides a measurement of approximately 12 normal minerals in the body, and most importantly, can detect the presence of toxic metals. It is a technique in which nutrient mineral element excesses or deficiencies in the body can be detected earlier than can be detected in the blood. Hair analysis is a relatively convenient and inexpensive procedure that requires about two tablespoons of hair.

The measured values of the minerals found in the hair may not always agree with whose found in blood. However, hair mineral analysis appears to be closely correlated with the mineral measurements made in bone.

Some researchers may argue that hair analysis measurements of the lighter elements, such as sodium and potassium, may contain some margin of error. However, the heavier the element, the less the margin of error and the more reliable the measurement. The heavier mineral elements such as the toxic metals can be measured accurately. In fact, hair mineral analysis has gained widespread use and respect as a technique for assessing body burdens of the heavy toxic metals. Some of these include lead, mercury, cadmium, aluminum, and copper. As environmental pollution increases, the load of these heavy metals building up in individuals is also likely to increase. Since heavy metal toxicity tends to affect the levels and ratios of important nutrient minerals in the tissues, the assessment of heavy toxic metals becomes extremely important. Hair mineral analysis has become increasingly useful for these assessments of heavy metal toxicity. The laboratory equipment and technology is now well developed for carrying out the needed chemical analyses with great precision. The same analytic techniques used for measuring heavy toxic metals in the hair also can be applied with precision for measuring essential nutrient minerals.

With the development of hair mineral analysis as a laboratory technique, a great deal of controversy has surfaced about some aspects of it. The major controversy has to do with the nutritional body correlates of essential nutrient minerals found in the hair. More specifically, can nutritional excesses and deficiencies be determined by means of a hair mineral analysis? Also, can an individual's need for vitamins and minerals be determined by this technique?

The basic questions relating hair mineral analysis to the nutritional status and needs of individuals require a conceptual system for interpreting the data found in the hair analysis chart. In order to make any sense of hair mineral analysis lab results, it is necessary to have a conceptual frame of reference for a meaningful interpretation. When hair nutrient mineral patterns are related to oxidation types (Watson, 1972) and the stages of the stress response (Selye, 1976) and its dynamics, especially involving the neuroendocrine system, these mineral patterns take on a great deal of psychological and physiological meaning.

Given the fact that the body's biochemistry involves a complex interaction of many vitamins, minerals, hormones, enzymes, etc., there is a dynamic, constantly changing chemical system regulating both physiological and psychological functions. The hair mineral analysis enables one to observe and to monitor some of the essential components of this dynamic system. Eck (1981) has described several of these patterns and interrelationships. He states that hair mineral ratios of Ca/K and Na/Mg could be used to determine oxidation types. This researcher also describes how these minerals and their ratios relate to Selye's three stages of the stress response. A significantly elevated sodium level is an index of aldosterone activity and, therefore, suggests that the individual has recently experienced the alarm stage of stress. When both sodium and potassium are significantly elevated in the hair mineral analysis, this reflects the resistance stage of stress. The increase in the potassium level serves as an index of glucocorticoid activity. And, finally, when both sodium and potassium levels fall significantly low, especially in relationship to calcium and magnesium, this is the exhaustion stage of stress. The first two stages of stress, alarm and resistance, tend to be conditions of fast oxidation, whereas the exhaustion stage tends to be the condition of slow oxidation.

The hair mineral analysis helps to identify a person's oxidation type. Fast oxidation is associated with hyperactivity of the major energy producing glands of the body, namely, the adrenals and the thyroid. Fast oxidation also tends to be associated with dominance of the sympathetic nervous system. Slow oxidation is associated with dominance of the parasympathetic nervous system. The ratio of calcium to potassium tends to be an index of thyroid activity, whereas the ratio of sodium to magnesium tends to be an index of adrenal activity.

In addition to determining the oxidation type from the hair tissue mineral analysis, the degree of fast or slow oxidation can also be determined. Thus, the ratios will be indices of the rate of oxidation. One may be designated a very fast oxidizer or a slightly fast oxidizer. Similarly, one may designate a person as a very slow oxidizer or a slightly slow oxidizer.

One of the most important concepts formulated by Eck for the interpretation of hair analysis data is the inversion of the Na/K ratio. When this ratio inverts (i.e., drops below 2.5), there is likely to be an increase in the manifestation of psychological and/or physical problems. This phenomenon can best be understood in terms of the role of sodium and potassium in cellular metabolism and the physiology of stress (Asterita, 1985). The Na/K ratio and its inversion is a critical ratio for both physiological and psychological functioning.

By relating hair mineral analysis results to the physiology of stress and oxidation types, it can be seen more clearly why the taking of some nutritional supplements may make a person worse, whereas the taking of other supplements may be very beneficial to the same person. For example, when a person is experiencing a Na/K inversion, then the taking of a zinc supplement usually makes the person worse simply because zinc raises potassium and lowers sodium in the tissues. This would result in lowering the Na/K ratio even more. Thus, it can be clearly seen that zinc functions as an anti-stress and anti-inflammatory mineral. Zinc is most useful in the presence of an elevated Na/K ratio because of its anti-stress and anti-inflammatory effect.

One of the most important principles related to a meaningful interpretation of a hair mineral analysis has to do with the fact that the hair analysis is a cross-section of a dynamic interacting system whose mineral patterns change over a period of time. Therefore, cross-sectional studies of hair mineral analyses can be very limited and/or misleading. For example, some individuals may have a "hidden" high copper or other heavy toxic metal which tests low in the first hair analysis. It is only over a period of time, usually after a person has gone on a corrective nutritional program, that excess copper which has been tightly bound up in tissue storage is eliminated and tests high in a subsequent hair analysis.

Another important principle related to the use of hair mineral analysis for developing a nutritional program for an individual has to do with drawing inferences about vitamins from the tissue mineral patterns. Since copper tends to destroy vitamin B_6, copper toxic individuals usually will need substantial B_6 supplementation. When a low sodium level is observed in a slow oxidizer, there is usually a substantial deficiency of vitamin C, vitamin E, and the B vitamins.

Hair analysis has recently been used in many criminal investigations, because an individual's diet, environment, and metabolism create a unique hair chemistry (analogous to fingerprints).

In summary, hair tissue mineral analysis may provide essential data on the underlying biochemistry of nutrient minerals and heavy toxic metals which affect a person's psychophysiological functions. When carefully interpreted and related to the physiology of stress, the hair mineral analysis can be an extremely valuable clinical tool. Hair analysis is a new technology definitely worth exploring for use in nutritional science. It certainly provides a new tool in the field of preventive health care. For a more detailed discussion, see Malter (1984–85), and Passwater and Cranton (1983).

8

OTHER NUTRIENTS

The primary sources of energy for the body come from carbohydrates, fats, and proteins. All of these nutrients are extremely important because they supply the necessary fuel and energy needed by the body to carry on its many daily functions.

PROTEINS

Proteins form an important class of substances necessary for life. Next to water, they are the most abundant substances found in the body which is composed of approximately 20 percent protein. Like carbohydrates and fats, they contain the elements carbon, hydrogen, and oxygen, but differ from carbohydrates and fats in that they contain nitrogen as well. Other constitutents of proteins are sulphur and sometimes iron, iodine, and phosphrous. Proteins essentially are composed of large numbers of amino acids, each amino acid linked to the next by a peptide bond. Although hundreds of amino acids exist in the body, there are approximately 20 amino acids that are commonly found in proteins and that have been identified as playing an important role in the several cellular processes. Of the 20 required amino acids, 12 of them are produced within the body. These amino acids are referred to as nonessential since the body does not have to rely upon specific food substances to produce them. The body independently manufactures them. These acids include:

alanine
arginine
asparagine
aspartic acid
cysteine
glutamine
glutamic acid
glycine

histidine
proline
serine
tyrosine

On the other hand, there is a group of eight amino acids that are not manufactured by the body and are indispensable for life. They are referred to as essential amino acids and can be obtained from specific food sources. These amino acids include:

isoleucine
leucine
lysine
methionine

phenylalanine
threonine
tryptophan
valine

Arginine and histidine are considered to be essential amino acids during the early years of child development since the body does not appear to manufacture them in adequate amounts as needed during the process of growing. These amino acids are not considered essential for adults.

During the process of digestion, proteins are broken down into amino acids. These amino acids are necessary for the synthesis of many body proteins. Not all of the proteins contain all the essential amino acids. Those proteins that do supply a proper balance of the essential amino acids are referred to as complete proteins (those found in fresh milk, egg yolk, wheat germ, etc). Those proteins that do not supply the body with an adequate amount of essential amino acids are termed incomplete (those found in grains, beans, peas, seeds, etc.). However, it is possible to form complete proteins from food that contains two or more incomplete proteins provided these proteins are eaten together. Some foods, such as seafood, cheese, and meats, do contain complete protein but the amount of essential amino acids are too small. Hence for a proper protein balance it is important to have a mixture of complete and incomplete proteins in the diet.

Proteins can probably be considered the most important nutrients in the body. They play an integral role in several chemical reactions, including hormone synthesis, acid base balance, and water balance. They are involved in several vital processes including growth, development, and repair of body tissue, digestion, elimination, and resistance to disease and infection. Enzymes, which are necessary for several vital functions, and antibodies, which help combat the invasion of foreign substances in the body, are both derived from protein sources. Proteins are also an important source of energy and the most important source of nitrogen.

There is an important relationship between proteins and sugar. The oxidation of sugar supplies the body with needed energy. Each cell requires sugar as a nutrient, and the amount of sugar in the blood is a determining factor for the sugar requirement of each cell. The metabolism or breakdown of protein supplies a certain percentage of this sugar. The presence of an adequate amount of protein regulates the digestive process so that sugar enters the circulation at a slower rate, thus maintaining a sustained level of energy.

Protein requirements vary and are a function of several factors, such as age, weight, and state of health. Naturally, the younger and larger you are, the greater the requirement of protein. The Recommended Dietary Allowance (RDA) per day of protein, in general, ranges from 23 to 36 grams for children, 44 to 54 grams for adolescents, and 48 to 56 grams for adults. In addition, it is recommended that pregnant women ingest an additional 30 grams and lactating women an additional 20 grams of protein per day.

Deficiency Disorders

Protein deficiency can lead to an impairment of tissue development and growth disorders. Severe protein deficiency in children results in an often fatal disease called kwashiorkor, which is accompanied by mental retardation and abnormalities in growth. In adults, protein deficiency may produce symptoms of mental depression, fatigue, weakness, a decrease in immune responsiveness, slow healing of wounds, and fluid imbalance.

Proteins and Stress

Some studies describe the changes in serum protein as a result of various types of stress exposure. Tollersrud et al. (1971) report a decrease in serum protein as a result of the stress of transport and herding in sheep. John and George (1977) describe the effect of heat stress in the pigeon and report a decrease in total serum protein and albumin. Wohler (1972) describes shipping stress in feeding cattle and the effect on total serum protein levels. Wohler found total serum protein levels to be generally depressed in various types of cattle one week after shipment. The protein levels had begun to normalize two weeks after arrival but remained below normal levels 75 days after shipment.

In general, several types of stress are known to result in a loss of protein from the body and produce a negative nitrogen balance. Such stresses include hemorrhage, surgical wounds, and chronic illnesses. As a result of several types of stress, there is an increase in glucocorticoid hormone production, which enhances the metabolism not only of proteins but also carbohydrates and fats. The increase in metabolism of these nutrients produces instant energy for the body, which is needed in times of stress. As a result of this, protein levels may decrease and some protein may be lost from the body.

During such types of stress exposure, it is important to include extra protein in the diet to replace the lost protein and to provide the necessary raw materials for protein synthesis, which may be needed for repair and the rebuilding of old, worn-out tissue.

Amino Acids and Stress

Certain essential and nonessential amino acids have been claimed to be effective in the management of stress. They are arginine, cystine and cysteine, *gamma*-aminobutyric acid (GABA), ornithine, and glutamic acid.

Cystine and cysteine are sulfur-containing essential amino acids (actually one amino acid is involved, existing in two forms) that exert an important protective effect on the body against various environmental pollutants. Sulfur acts as an antioxidant, which can protect the body against oxidation. Sulfur, through its antioxidative effects, can deactivate free radicals, neutralize toxins, and therefore protect against cellular and tissue damage. Cystine and cysteine act in this capacity and therefore serve as protective agents for the body against several environmental chemical stresses, including such common ones as smog and tobacco smoke. When cystine and cysteine are combined with vitamin E, the total antioxidant effect is enhanced. A combination of these substances can help prevent unnecessary fat catabolism in the body since uncontrolled fat breakdown can result in the release of free radicals. Free radical formation that results from normal metabolic processes and oxidation in the body must be controlled, otherwise tissue damage and premature aging may occur.

Gamma-aminobutyric acid, an amino acid derivative, is an important brain neurotransmitter. Some studies report that *gamma*-aminobutyric acid in combination with inositol and niacinamide acts as an antianxiety agent, thereby functioning to combat stress. This particular combination of *gamma*-aminobutyric acid and the B vitamins has been claimed to have a relaxing and tranquilizing effect on the body.

Arginine and ornithine are two amino acids that either when acting alone or combined can enhance the anterior pituitary gland to secrete growth hormone. The secretion of growth hormone is generally increased as a result of the elicitation of the stress response, particularly chronic stress. It is known that growth hormone has a stimulating effect on the immune system and in this sense exerts a protective effect on the body during times of stress. It does this by enhancing the destruction of any bacteria, viruses, or foreign toxins that may have invaded the body. Arginine and ornithine, therefore, indirectly enhance the functioning of the immune system through their effect on growth hormone secretion.

Other amino acids that can be considered to play a role in counteracting stress include phenylalanine, tyrosine, tryptophan, glutamic acid, histidine, and methionine. Phenylalanine and tyrosine are well known for their mood elevation properties and may play an important role in the treatment of various anxiety states and sleep disorders. In the brain, tryptophan is converted into the neurotransmitter serotonin, and it is well known that serotonin is involved in proper brain functioning and mental health. Individuals who suffer depression or insomnia have low levels of serotónin.

Glutamic acid can be helpful in times of stress by being instrumental in increasing the supply of energy to brain cells. Some reports in the literature indicate that glutamic acid and glutamine supplementation have produced positive results in the cognitive processes of learning and memory when used in conjunction with therapy in the treatment of mental illnesses in the elderly.

Histidine, another amino acid worth mentioning, may also be important in times of stress, particularly in allergic reactions. Allergies appear to be a stress-related disorder, and allergy attacks appear to be exacerbated in times of stress. Some reports claim that histidine may be effective in allergy treatment. In conditions of stress, trauma, or shock, histamine is generally released by the soft tissues of the body. Some studies indicate that histamine levels decrease as the levels of histidine are increased in the body through dietary means.

Although there are some indications that a relationship may exist between histidine and allergic reactions, further work is required to clarify any possible role this amino acid may play in the overall stress response.

Methionine, an essential amino acid, may play a role in the body as an antistress amino acid. It appears to be important in cleansing the kidneys and the liver by aiding in the elimination of toxic waste products from these organs.

Although several of the amino acids have been implicated in playing a role in the elicitation of the stress response by acting in a positive manner, particularly as protective agents in the face of several types of stress exposure, the underlying physiological mechanisms involved remain to be clarified.

CARBOHYDRATES

Carbohydrates consist of a class of organic compounds composed mainly of carbon, hydrogen, and oxygen. The hydrogen and oxygen are combined in the same ratio as water and are bound (hydrated) to carbon, hence the name carbohydrates. The compounds are represented by the formula $C_x(H_2O)_y$. For example, glucose has the formula $C_6(H_2O)_6$ or $C_6H_{12}O_6$ and sucrose, $C_{12}H_{22}O_{11}$.

Although the body is composed of approximately 12 percent carbohydrate, these compounds make up the major part of the diet, and are thus the main source of energy in most nations of the world. They constitute 45 to 50 percent of the daily caloric intake in developed nations and approximately 90 percent in developing nations.

Carbohydrates consist not only of sugars but also of starches. All carbohydrates are broken down into the simple sugar glucose, which is a measure of blood sugar in the circulating blood. Glucose is an important nutrient for all the cells of the body, in particular for the central nervous system. Carbohydrates aid in the regulation of protein and fat metabolism. It is important to have an adequate intake of carbohydrates so that the body need not resort to proteins as an energy source. It is much more important for proteins to be used in the vital processes of tissue building and repair rather than as a main source of energy. Also, fats required the presence of carbohydrates for their breakdown in the liver.

Carbohydrates, which the body does not use immediately, are stored in the liver and muscle in the form of glycogen. Carbohydrates taken into the body, in excess of the storage capacity for glycogen, are converted into fat. The more carbohydrate that is converted to fat, the more weight is gained. When the body needs more energy to carry on with its various functions, the fat is converted back to glucose and weight is lost.

There is no official Recommended Dietary Allowance for carbohydrates. However, it is thought that a minimum of 50 grams daily should be part of the diet. The general trend today is that Americans in general eat far too many carbohydrates and therefore tend to be prone to gaining weight.

Carbohydrates are found in most of our food sources with the exception of meats, fats, oils, and a small number of other nutrient foods.

Carbohydrates and Stress

In the face of various types of stress exposure, the need is often to acquire more energy. To achieve this, many individuals have formed the habit of eating snacks containing sugars and starches. Such foods do provide the body with instant energy because they allow the blood sugar level to increase suddenly. With the sudden increase in blood sugar, there is also a subsequent rapid fall of blood sugar. The desire for more of such foods then increases. This eventually could lead to weakness, fatigue, headache, and nervousness.

If such carbohydrates are taken in excess, a nutritional deficiency can result. Since excess carbohydrate is converted into fat in the body, overweight and obesity can also occur. A diet of refined carbohydrates is generally low in vitamins, minerals, and fiber. In particular, if such a diet is maintained, a B vitamin deficiency is likely to ensue, which in turn is an added source of stress to the body. Perhaps such stress-related disorders as diabetes, heart disease, high blood pressure, and even cancer may be related in some way to an excessive amount of dietary refined carbohydrates.

Glucose and Stress

Several studies describe the effects of various types of stress exposure on carbohydrate metabolism and blood sugar levels.

Kameyama et al. (1981) describe the environmental stress of high temperature and humidity on blood glucose levels of laboratory mice. They report that blood glucose levels increase upon a short-term exposure to stress and decrease with a long-term exposure. The mice exhibit adaptation during chronic stress exposure.

The adrenal cortex, through its synthesis and secretion of the glucocorticoids, plays a role in regulating plasma levels of glucose. The adrenal cortex is highly sensitive to various types of stress exposure. Kameyama et al. (1981) suggest that the initial transient increase in blood glucose as a result of the stress response may be related to a release of epinephrine in the first stage of the alarm reaction. The ensuing state of hypoglycemia may be due to a subsequent relative hypofunction of the adrenal cortex and a decrease in glucocorticoid production, in accordance with Selye's later stages of the general adaptation syndrome. Kameyama et al. (1981) also investigated substances such as pantothenic acid (vitamin B_5) and ascorbic acid (vitamin C), among others, which are known to influence the adrenal gland. They found that the administration of pantothenic acid, a substance known to enhance adrenal activity, tended to inhibit the stress-induced hypoglycemia, while both acute and chronic administration of ascorbic acid significantly inhibited hypoglycemia in stressed animals.

Arola et al. (1980) describe the change in several plasma metabolites when laboratory animals were exposed to a mild form of stress. They found a significant decrease in the size of the liver as well as glycogen content along with a fall in plasma insulin and a rise in the levels of blood glucose as a result of mild stress exposure. Arola et al. report a significant fall in blood lactate in the stressed group of animals. Their study also describes differences in blood composition of metabolities at different sampling sites.

Steyn (1975) studied the effect of captivity stress on blood glucose in baboons and observed an initial decrease followed by a significant increase in blood sugar levels.

Tigranian et al. (1980), in their investigative work on the changes that take place in many of the blood nutrients in male students undergoing the emotional stress of an academic examination, found blood glucose levels to be within a normal range before the examination. After the examination, however, they found a significant increase in blood glucose levels. A significant increase in growth hormone secretion and in insulin secretion was also observed. Growth hormone and insulin have opposite effects on blood glucose (growth hormone raising and insulin lowering it). These researchers suggest that the changes observed in these hormones and blood glucose levels may reflect a glycolysis inhibition and an enhancement of gluconeogenesis, both of which result in an increase in blood glucose levels.

Other researchers have reported similar results on emotional stress exposure (Dolkas et al. 1971). Hall and Brown (1979) studied the fluctuations in plasma glucose and lactate levels in subjects at four different periods during an examination. They found plasma glucose to be significantly elevated during a preexam period. Glucose then decreased significantly from preexam to postexam periods. On the other hand, lactate was significantly increased during preexam and increased significantly from preexam to postexamination. Hall and Brown hold that the condition of psychological stress results in a mobilization of glucose with a resulting increase in blood glucose levels. This increase in glucose feeds back to the pancreas and insulin secretion is enhanced, which, in turn, increases the uptake of glucose into muscle cells. In muscle, glucose is converted to lactic acid. Hence the postexam period is characterized by a significant decrease in blood glucose and a significant increase in blood lactate. Reilly and Chandrasena (1979) also report a rise in blood lactate in experimental sheep before the onset of a stress exposure (anticipatory stress).

The sugar concentration in the blood obtained from normal persons who have fasted for 12 hours lies in the range of 90 to 95 milligrams per 100 cubic centimeters of blood. This is the average level for blood sugar and is adequate for energy production. When blood sugar levels fall below this level to approximately 70 milligrams per 100 cubic centimeters of blood, symptoms of hypoglycemia appear. Such symptoms include muscular weakness, fatigue, and sometimes headache and nausea. States of hypoglycemia stress the body. Hypoglycemia in turn can result from the stress response itself, mediated through endocrine hormonal changes and several other biochemical and physiological factors. In any event, changes in blood sugar occur as a result of the elicitation of the stress response. These changes may be acute or chronic, depending on the nature of the stress response.

In summary, blood glucose levels generally appear to increase as a result of the presence of acute or intense stress. Other reports describe either no change or a decrease in blood glucose levels as a result of the stress response. The differing results reflect the multiple factors involved in the regulation of blood glucose levels. Some factors involved in the stress-induced changes in blood glucose levels are the nutritional state of the organism, the presence of other nutrients in the circulation, the secretion of other stress hormones, many of which enhance blood sugar levels, insulin levels, and the activity of the autonomic nervous system.

Cortisol, epinephrine, growth hormone, glucagon, and prolactin generally all increase in the circulation as a result of the stress response, and all of these hormones are known to enhance blood sugar levels. Insulin, on the other hand, is generally depressed as a result of the stress response.

The autonomic nervous system influences blood sugar levels. The parasympathetic system stimulates pancreatic insulin secretion. Insulin promotes the transport of glucose into cells, thereby decreasing blood glucose levels. Insulin also promotes the storage of sugar in the form of glycogen in both the liver and muscle. If blood sugar levels remain low for a period of time, fatigue, drowsiness, and lethargy appear as common symptoms. The activation of the sympathetic portion of the autonomic nervous system, as usually occurs with elicitation of the stress response, results in the adrenal medullary secretion of the catecholamines. The catecholamine, epinephrine, enhances glycogenolysis, which is the breakdown of glycogen, and therefore promotes the release of the stored glucose into the circulation, raising blood glucose levels. Since blood sugar is elevated, more of this nutrient is available to cells as the metabolism is increased. There is a sharpening of mental processes and more energy is available for use in states of emergency and stress.

To summarize, the net effect concerning the changes which occur in blood glucose levels as a result of stress, is a function of several factors, and in the final analysis, depends on the physiological state of the organism. Blood sugar levels could very well return to normal as stress adaptation takes place, but again, several factors related to the stress situation could override the return of blood glucose levels back to normal.

FATS

Fats, or lipids, are a class of compounds, like carbohydrates, that contain carbon, hydrogen, and oxygen, but not as much oxygen. Fats occur in nature generally combined with protein and carbohydrates. They are found in both plants and animals. Fats are not soluble in water but are soluble in ether, benzene, and other organic fat solvents.

In the fat molecule itself, one molecule of glycerol (an alcohol) is combined with three molecules of fatty acids forming a triglyceride. Many fatty acids are available in the body, but palmitic acid ($C_{18}H_{32}O_2$), oleic acid ($C_{18}H_{34}O_2$), and stearic acid ($C_{18}H_{36}O_2$) provide the largest quantities. There are also three "essential" fatty acids in the body. These are collectively known as vitamin F (see Chapter 4).

In the digestive process, fats are broken down (hydrolyzed) into fatty acids and glycerol. Glycerol and fatty acids then enter the epithelial cells, where they recombine to form neutral fats that then enter the blood-stream. Fatty acids are necessary for the growth and maintenance of the organism. Fatty acids give fats their different flavors, textures, and melting points.

Fatty acids are of two types: saturated or unsaturated. Unsaturated fatty acids, including the polyunsaturates, are derived from vegetables, nuts, and seeds and are liquid at room temperature. Substances containing unsaturated fatty acids are natural vegetable oils (corn, safflower, peanut, etc.), wheat germ, mayonnaise, sunflower seeds, nuts, and olives. Substances that contain saturated fatty acids are derived primarily from animal sources (except coconut oil) and include fatty meats, butter, and cream.

Although the body is composed of approximately 15 percent fat under normal conditions the body uses fats in several ways. When fats are oxidized, they are an important source of energy. Fats are used to support many organs, such as the kidneys, heart, liver, and eyes. Fat forms a protective sheath for muscles and nerves. In addition, fat forms an important component of the cell membrane of all cells of the body. Fats also reside in subcutaneous structures and form an insulating layer, thus conserving body heat and body temperature. Fats are necessary for normal growth and help keep the skin healthy and youthful through lubrication. The presence of fat is necessary for the absorption of the fat-soluble vitamins, A, D, E, and K.

By aiding in the absorption of vitamin D, fats aid in the use of calcium, which is so necessary for bones and teeth. Like carbohydrates, fats help conserve the use of protein for energy. A reserve of fat can be an important source of energy, particularly in an inadequate diet. Fats have a high caloric value, particularly when compared to carbohydrates and proteins. When oxidized, fats yield almost twice as many calories as carbohydrates or proteins. Fats yield approximately 9 calories per gram while carbohydrates and proteins each yield approximately half of that value.

To date, no dietary recommended allowance has been established for fats. However, taking more than an adequate amount of fat into the body can lead to overweight, heart disease, and other clinical disorders.

Deficiency Conditions

Humans rarely experience a deficiency in fat. Should one occur, it would result in a deficiency of the fat-soluble vitamins. Various skin disorders and growth retardation can occur in cases of severe deficiency.

Free Fatty Acids and Stress

Stress-induced stimulation of the sympathetic–adrenal medullary axis leads to elevated circulating levels of the catecholamines, norepine-phrine and epinephrine (Euler, 1964). Elevated plasma levels of the catecholamines result in an increase in their urinary excretion (Levi 1963), which often serves as a measure of the stress response.

The free fatty acids (FFA) from adipose tissue are mobilized in the presence of the catecholamines (Havel and Goldfien 1959). Catech-olamine-induced FFA mobilization from adipose tissue results in elevated levels of triglycerides in the liver (Feigelson et al. 1961). Triglyceride elevations in the liver, in turn, result in a release of these metabolites into the circulation, with a consequent rise in plasma triglycerides (Friedman and Byers 1960). During stress, the energy demand is increased, and the elevated free fatty acids in the circulation can serve as a needed source for energy. Several researchers have observed elevations in circulating FFA during short-term arousal in humans and animals (Gordon and Gordon 1959; Kahn et al. 1964; Mayes 1962).

In particular, Reynaert et al. (1976) demonstrate that stress provokes a significant increase in free fatty acids in cattle. Benes and Hrubes (1968) describe a study in which the serum FFA were determined in laboratory animals before and after one hour of stress exposure to intermittent electric shocks. The FFA levels in serum increased in stressed animals. The group of animals that demonstrated a small degree of adaptation exhibited even higher levels of FFA after stress.

In both animal and human studies, the blood levels of free fatty acids are invariably increased by several types of stress exposure (Chait et al. 1979; Taggart and Carruthers 1971; Taggart et al. 1973; Carlson et al. 1968; Dimsdale and Herd 1982; Gittleman et al. 1968; Gordon and Gordon 1959; Bogdonoff et al. 1959). Several studies show that plasma lipids are greatly influenced by short-term emotional arousal (Dimsdale and Herd 1982).

Mueller et al. (1970) found elevated plasma free fatty acid concentrations in severely depressed patients, and Valek and Kuln (1970) demonstrate a higher sensitivity of lipid metabolism in coronary heart disease patients to the stressful stimuli of everyday life.

Another lipid constituent of plasma includes the triglycerides (a molecule of three fatty acids linked to glycerol, as described earlier). Researchers have found no consistent pattern of triglyceride response to emotional stress (Dimsdale and Herd 1982). Acute stress has been shown to either increase, decrease, or have little or no effect on plasma triglycerides (Chait et al. 1979). In addition, Chait et al. demonstrate a lowering of plasma triglyceride concentration as a result of three different forms of acute stress in humans.

Perhaps these conflicting data may be a result of a failure to distinguish acute from chronic stress, the variation in intensity with which the stressful stimulus is perceived, as well as a lack of control with regard to the dietary states of the subjects.

In general, the free fatty acid levels and other lipids such as cholesterol all appear to be elevated in the circulation as a result of several types of stress exposure. Triglyceride levels are also generally elevated as a result of stress, although several studies do not confirm such a view.

CHOLESTEROL

Cholesterol belongs to the group of nutrients known as the lipids. Its presence in the body is necessary for the maintenace of health. The molecular formula of cholesterol is that of a monohydric alcohol ($C_{27}H_{45}OH$).

Cholesterol is probably the most common animal sterol (unsaturated solid alcohol of the steroid group) and is found in all tissues especially in blood cells, bile, plasma, the kidney, the liver (where it is synthesized), the intestine, and nervous tissue (brain and spinal cord). It plays an important role in the synthesis of various steroid hormones and metabolic processes, particularly carbohydrate metabolism.

Cholesterol acts as a precursor in the formation of bile salts, vitamin D, and the synthesis of various steroid hormones, such as the glucocorticoids and the sex hormones.

While it is a popular belief that cholesterol can be responsible for cardiovascular disease, arteriosclerosis, and a variety of illnesses, cholesterol is essential in the maintenance of a normal, healthy body. It is needed for the digestion of fats.

The effects of cholesterol in the body are varied and depend on which circulating lipoprotein cholesterol is bound to when it is transported in the circulation. Very low-density lipoproteins (VLDL) transport about 15 percent of the total amount of cholesterol. This fraction appears to correlate well with cardiovascular disorders. Low-density lipoproteins (LDL), also implicated in cardiovascular disease, contain a small amount of protein and transport approximately 20 percent of the cholesterol. The HDL fraction appears to have an effect opposite to that of the LDL and VLDL. HDL appears to play an active role in protecting the body against cardiovascular disease. HDL appears to transport cholesterol without resulting in the buildup of plaque and the clogging up of arteries, which increases the risk of stroke and heart attack. HDL contains lecithin, which possesses detergent like activity and which, in turn, acts to break up cholesterol molecules without causing subsequent arterial damage. It therefore appears that the higher the LDL fraction, the greater the chances are for developing heart disease, and the greater the HDL fraction, the less the chances are for developing heart disease. In other words, high-density lipoproteins have an inverse relationship to the risk of developing coronary artery disease (Painter et al. 1972).

A diet rich in saturated fatty acids (meats and dairy products) increases blood cholesterol levels, while a diet rich in unsaturated fatty acids (vegetables and fish) results in a somewhat lower level of cholesterol.

Some of the foods containing cholesterol are egg yolk, milk, and several types of animal fats and oils. As yet, no correlation between egg consumption and heart disease has been demonstrated. Although eggs are thought to be hazardous to health, they can actually play a positive role in health maintenance. Eggs contain practically the best protein components of any food substance and, most of all, they contain lecithin, which helps in the assimilation of fats by the body. Eggs result in an increase in HDL rather than an increase in LDL levels in the bloodstream.

Epidemiological studies point to a strong relationship between cholesterol and saturated fat in the diet and the prevalence of cardiovascular disease (Feldman 1976; Keys 1970). Diet and the high circulating levels of blood lipids, particularly cholesterol and saturated fat, play a role in the development of atherosclerosis. Not only the risk but also the development and the progression of cardiovascular disease appear to be associated with cholesterol levels higher than 250 milligrams/100 milliliters. The blood levels of cholesterol depend partially on the dietary intake of cholesterol and saturated and polyunsatured fats. Dietary saturated fats tend to increase plasma cholesterol levels while polyunsaturated fats tend to decrease cholesterol levels (Feldman 1976; Dayton 1976). Populations that have low levels of cholesterol and saturated fat in their diet have low plasma cholesterol levels and a small incidence of coronary heart disease, although, there are some exceptions to this rule. Many researchers today think that increasing the HDL-cholesterol fraction in the blood through diet should result in a decreased progression of atherosclerosis. Some evidence does exist that a regression in arterial damage has occurred in some patients after dietary treatment. Dietary factors that are known to influence plasma lipids and decrease plasma cholesterol levels are protein, certain kinds of fiber, vitamin D, calcium, vanadium, silicate, and the zinc-copper ratio.

The Recommended Daily Allowance of cholesterol for the average person is considered to be no more than 300 milligrams.

Several factors other than diet have been shown to raise cholesterol levels in the blood. Two such factors are cigarette smoking and exercise. There are indications that nonsmokers have higher HDL concentrations than smokers and that athletes have a higher concentration of HDL than less physically active people.

Other nondietary factors that may play a role in raising cholesterol levels include oral contraceptives, coffee, alcohol, and refined sugar.

Cholesterol and Stress

Various types of stress exposure have been shown to elevate blood cholesterol levels in laboratory animals. Rothfeld et al. (1970) demonstrate that cholesterol levels are increased in various tissues of stressed laboratory rats fed a high cholesterol diet compared to unstressed animals fed a similar diet. These researchers report an increase in cholesterol in the serum, aorta, and liver along with a mild transient elevation in the kidneys of the stressed animals. In a later work, Paré et al. (1973) and Rothfeld et al. (1973) subjected rats fed a high-fat diet to the psychological stress of unpredictable and uncontrollable foot shock over a specified time period. Their results confirm earlier data in which higher cholesterol levels were found in the serum of tissues of stressed animals than in control animals, both of which were fed a high-fat diet. Similar work is reported by Berger et al. (1980), who subjected laboratory rats to either the stress of predictable and controllable (escape/avoidance) foot shock, the stress of unpredictable and uncontrollable foot shock, or no foot shock (unstressed). They found the plasma cholesterol levels to be higher in the unpredictable and uncontrollable stressed treatment group. The plasma cholesterol levels were also higher for the shocked stressed animals than the unshocked (unstressed) animals.

Research that has focused on stressful life situations also demonstrates an elevation of plasma cholesterol during stress exposure (Sloane et al. 1961; Cathey et al. 1957; Henry et al. 1971).

Chronic stress exposure in humans has been shown by other researchers to lead to elevations in plasma concentrations of cholesterol (Mann and White 1953; Thomas and Murphy 1958; Friedman et al. 1958; Grundy and Griffin 1959a; Dreyfuss and Czaczkes 1959; Wertlake et al. 1968) and to low-density lipoproteins (Grundy and Griffin 1959b; Francis 1979). Also many studies indicate that cholesterol increases from 8 to 65 percent above baseline levels under conditions of stress (Dimsdale and Herd 1982).

The serum levels of cholesterol are under hormonal influence. In particular, the excess glucocorticoids present in the circulation as a result of stress may very well influence cholesterol levels and other lipids (Mann and White 1953). Cholesterol is a precursor substance in the steroidogenesis of adrenal hormones. The elevated serum cholesterol level may indeed serve the purpose of being a potential source of steroid synthesis during times of stress, or it may serve other purposes (Francis 1979). The mechanisms involved in the sustained elevations in serum cholesterol as a result of stress are open for further study.

OTHER METABOLIC FACTORS

Several other metabolites are very necessary for normal physiological functioning. Some of these factors are involved in normal metabolic processes and some of them have been shown to be influenced by the stress response.

URIC ACID

Uric acid is a urinary product of purine metabolism derived from nucleoproteins. Its only known route of exit from the body is through the urine. Uric acid levels are increased in the urine during ingestion of proteins and other nitrogen-containing foods. Also, elevated uric acid levels have been known to occur after exercise in people with leukemia, gout, and acute articular rheumatism. Recently, it has been shown that there is an association between serum uric acid levels and certain types of human behavior patterns that are linked to the perception and/or experience of stress.

Uric acid is chemically related to the stimulants caffeine and theophylline, and it may therefore act as an endogenously produced stimulant for the central nervous system. Perhaps, as the serum level of uric acid changes as a result of stress exposure, its stimulant activity on the central nervous system is modified accordingly.

Uric Acid and Stress

Some studies demonstrate that serum uric acid levels appear to be associated with stress exposure. Uric acid levels may be correlated with an individual's successful handling of a stressful confrontation. Rahe et al. (1968) and Brooks and Mueller (1966) have described high serum uric acid levels associated with people who are hardworking, successful, of leadership quality, and who experience life situations more as challenges, leading toward achievement, than as stressful events. On the other hand, a lowering of serum uric acid levels has been found by some researchers to occur when individuals anticipate life situations as stressful and feel overloaded, tense, nervous, anxious, hostile, and depressed (Rahe et al. 1968; Rahe et al. 1971; Francis 1979). Francis reports serum uric acid levels to be significantly depressed in students during the first half of an academic quarter and a return to control levels after midterm exams. Rahe et al. (1968, 1971) report a decrease in serum uric acid levels in United States naval personnel during the initial training period of "Hellweek" at the underwater demolition training school. In an earlier study, Rahe and Arthur (1967) demonstrate higher than normal levels of uric acid (6.5 milligrams/100 milliliters as compared to 4.9 milligrams/100 milliliters) in naval personnel during their experience of "Hellweek" at the underwater demolition training school.

In addition, an earlier study by Hoffel and Moriarty (1924) demonstrates high uric acid levels in children undergoing the stress of starvation during a period of six to nine days. It is thought that stress along with the acidotic condition produced in this nutritionally deficient state may both contribute to the rise in uric acid levels.

Pregnancy has been shown to be accompanied by an elevation in serum uric acid levels that is maintained for many weeks postpartum. (Pfeiffer et al. 1969) Pfeiffer et al. also demonstrate that schizophrenic patients have a higher degree of serum uric acid levels on entering the hospital than when they were discharged after their psychosis was treated. These researchers state that the level of serum uric acid may be an indication of the degree of stress experienced by the schizophrenic patients since the serum uric acid levels appear to decrease with antipsychotic therapy.

Several other studies demonstrate higher levels of uric acid in certain population groups. Dunn et al. (1963) report that in different male populations, executives have higher serum uric acid levels than craftsmen, Ph.D. researchers have higher levels than supervisors, supervisors have higher levels than craftsmen and medical students have higher uric acid levels than high school students. These and other studies indicate that serum uric acid levels appear to decrease during the stress of nervousness and anxiety (Francis 1979; Rahe et al. 1968; 1971), while uric acid levels are higher in those individuals who experience stress in times of achievement (Stetten 1959; Stetten and Hearon 1959). The underlying mechanisms involved in the stress-induced alteration of serum uric acid levels are not well known and need further clarification.

ENZYMES

Enzymes are composed of proteins. More than 650 of them are known. They are produced by living organisms, both plants and animals. They act as catalysts in the various chemical reactions that take place in the body. They generally speed up the rate of chemical reactions with which they are associated. Many enzymes require the aid of certain coenzymes to properly function in their biological roles. Most of the coenzymes are members of the vitamin B complex family.

Enzymes are particularly found in digestive juices, which aid in the breakdown of food into simpler substances. Hence they are necessary for digestion, which results not only in the breakdownn of proteins, carbohydrates, and fats, but also the release of various vitamins and minerals necessary for the healthy functioning of the body.

Enzymes are specific in their activity; they will act only on certain food substances or closely related substances and no other.

Enzymes are rendered inactive under high or low temperatures. Each enzyme has a particular temperature and pH in which it acts at optimum efficiency. Enzyme activity can be altered in the presence of ultraviolet radiation, dehydration, and heavy metals such as copper, mercury, and lead.

Enzymes are vital for all bodily processes. A deficiency of even one enzyme can cause illness.

Enzymes and Stress

Some studies in the literature describe the changes in enzyme activity as a result of stress.

Tollersrud (1969, 1970) and Tollersrud et al. (1971) demonstrate that enzyme levels increase in animals as a result of stress exposure. Tollersrud et al. (1971) describe the effect of transportation stress and physical activity in sheep on various serum enzymes. They observed elevated serum enzyme activity during transportation and subsequent herding of the animals. They suggest, along with others, that the increase in serum enzyme activity after physical exercise may be due to an increase in permeability of the cell membranes. This increase in membrane permeabililty may be due to an increase in endocrine hormonal activity induced by stress. Tollersrud et al. report that the greatest increase in serum enzyme activity occurred in lambs that were not used to physical exercise.

Steyn (1975), working with the Chacma baboon, found an increase in serum enzyme activity associated with the stress of captivity in these animals.

These few examples, as well as several other research reports in the literature, demonstrate a definite stress-induced increase in enzyme activity. The increase in several specific enzymes have also been reported by many researchers. The stress-induced alterations in enzyme activity may very well reflect the changes in metabolism and other physiological processes that occur as a result of various types of stress exposure.

WATER

Water, the universal solvent, is vital to the functioning of all body processes. It is without doubt the most important nutrient. More than 50 percent of all body tissues are composed of water. The body itself is composed of approximately 70–90 percent of water. Water is present in the fluid within the cells, the intracellular fluid, and in the fluid bathing the cells, the extracellular fluid. In addition, it is found in blood, lymph, gastric juice, bile, sweat, and urine.

Water is an absolutely essential intracellular medium where the metabolic processes and various other vital chemical reactions take place. Both within and outside cells, it is the medium in which acids and bases react to produce the necessary acid-base balance in the body. The establishment and maintenance of the necessary acid-base balance is vital for maintaining the proper concentrations of electrolytes and for promoting those essential ionization reactions that occur both inside and outside the cells. All of these factors contribute toward maintaining normal physiological balance, or homeostasis.

Water has a high specific heat and latent heat of vaporization. It therefore serves an important role in both the regulation and maintenance of a constant body temperature.

Water does not contain any nutrients or vitamins but does contain minerals and mineral salts. For example, magnesium and calcium are present in hard water, and specific mineral waters may contain silicates, chlorides and carbonates. Well water generally contains large amounts of iron.

Generally, the average healthy person ingests about 5½ pints of water daily. Approximately 3 pints come from the drinking of water alone and water-containing beverages such as coffee and soft drinks and 2½ pints come from solid foods such as vegetables and fruits and liquid foods such as milk and soup. Approximately 60 percent of the water ingested is eliminated as urine, 25 percent as perspiration through the pores of the skin, 12 percent is exhaled as water vapor through the lungs, and 3 percent is eliminated from the body in the feces.

There is no Recommended Dietary Allowance for water, since water intake and elimination are functions of factors such as climate and diet. However, water intake is generally dictated by thirst. About six glasses of water per day are recommended. Excessive water intake can lead to water intoxication while an excessive loss of water can lead to dehydration.

Water and Stress

Various types of stress exposures have been associated with an increase in water retention in the body. This water retention appears to be mediated through an increase in body sodium due in part to an enhanced stress-induced hormonal secretion of aldosterone. Several types of stress, including emotional stress, have also been shown to influence the secretion of antidiuretic hormone (ADH). An increase in ADH secretion occurs in response to stress, thereby contributing toward increased water retention by the body. The increased levels of both aldosterone and ADH as a result of stress contribute toward a definite sodium and water retention and can be viewed as an important adaptation response, particularly as a protective measure against losses incurred by sweating and hemorrhage.

9

SUPPLEMENTARY FOODS

While it is beyond the scope of this text to discuss the different well-known food groups in terms of various dietary regimens, mention is made here of some foods that may serve as adjunct nutrients in times of stress.

Some supplementary foods are now available on the market that may be included as part of the diet to increase the nutritional value of one's daily food intake. Many of these foods are available in convenient form, as tablets, powders, capsules, and liquids.

ACIDOPHILUS

Acidophilus is a source of intestinal bacteria and is available as a culture. Some researchers think that appropriate use of this culture will provide the intestinal tract with an adequate amount of intestinal flora and therefore maintain the intestines in a healthy condition. Fiber in the diet and complex carbohydrates are at least two other dietary sources that help the growth of intestinal bacteria. Taking acidophilus in appropriate amounts may eliminate such disorders as constipation (sometimes the result of acute or chronic stress).

ALFALFA

Alfalfa is a leguminous plant and is familiar in the form of seeds and sprouts. It is a very rich source of almost all of the vitamins, particularly vitamin K. It is also a good source of many minerals. Alfalfa contains several essential enzymes. In view of its nutrient value, alfalfa may well be a helpful adjunct to the diet in times of stress.

BEE PROPOLIS

Bee propolis is primarily composed of a resinous material that the bees produce and use in their hives. It is a natural antibiotic for them. Recent research, however, suggests its beneficial effects not only for bees but also for humans. Some researchers have found bee propolis to be effective in fighting both viral and bacterial infections in humans. In view of its claimed antiinfection properties, bee propolis may very well serve a positive role in times of intense stress by providing the body with the needed resistance to ward off any foreign or infectious agents.

BLACKSTRAP MOLASSES

Blackstrap molasses is a supplementary food that is a very rich source of both vitamins and minerals. Of the sugar products, it contains by far the most nutrients. Some researchers claim that many stress-related conditions, such as ulcers, constipation, and skin problems, may respond well by supplementing the diet with a daily small amount (one tablespoon) of this substance.

BONE MEAL

Bone meal is a supplementary food that consists of the finely ground bone of cattle. It is a good calcium and phosphorus source and contains trace minerals that promote the healthy development of bones and teeth.

BREWER'S YEAST

Brewer's yeast is one of the best sources of the B vitamins and several minerals. It also contains several amino acids. It may be a beneficial adjunct to the ordinary diet, particularly in times of stress.

DESICCATED LIVER

Desiccated liver is rich in vitamins A, C, and D and calcium, phosphorus, and iron. Desiccated liver may be combined with other foods to provide a rich source of vitamins and minerals.

TABLE 9.1 Fiber Types and Their Food Sources

Fiber Type	Food Source
Cellulose	Coarse bran, fresh carrots, unpeeled apples and pears
Hemicellulose	Bran cereals, whole grain breads
Lignin	Toasted whole grain breads, fried and brown potatoes
Pectin	Bananas, apples, potatoes, carrots, oranges
Gums	Oatmeal, sesame seeds

FIBER

Brief mention should be made of the importance of fiber in the diet. Although fiber is not a nutrient in the strict sense of the word, since it does not supply energy to the body, in a very real sense it plays an important role in human nutrition. In particular, recent research suggests an important role for dietary fiber in the process of digestion.

The content of proteins, fats, carbohydrates, vitamins, and minerals is the basis by which the nutritional quality of foods is generally judged. Fiber content of foods is also of importance, although it is not generally included along with these nutrients.

Fiber, or roughage (the indigestible parts of food), is important for the proper functioning of the digestive tract in promoting the elimination of wastes from the body. Fiber aids in the regularity of bowel movements. In addition, the presence of adequate amounts of fiber in the intestinal tract results in the absorption of large amounts of water, thus resulting in the softening of fecal material.

Dietary fiber also provides bulk material to the digestive tract without supplying energy. Hence, in a limited way, it can be used to reduce caloric intake.

The source of human dietary fiber is derived from plants. Fiber is composed of complex carbohydrates, which includes cellulose, found in the cell wall of all plant cells, lignin, pectin, and gums. The different types of fiber and their food sources are listed in Table 9.1.

Food sources of fiber include celery stalks, the stems of salad greens, vegetables, potatoes, raw fruits, fruits with whole grain seeds, cereals, and unprocessed bran. In general, unrefined foods contain more fiber than refined or processed foods. The fiber contained within these unrefined foods is not digested. As the food particles containing fiber move through the digestive tract, they absorb liquid and swell. They provide a large quantity of soft bulk to other materials found in the digestive tract, and as previously stated, result in an increase in bowel movement.

Many researchers today feel that it is of physiological benefit to have a good supply of fiber in the diet. They think that the intestinal activity resulting from fiber in the diet can decrease the amount of fat metabolities thought to be associated with colonic cancer. On the basis of epidemiological evidence, it appears that an insufficient amount of fiber in the diet can increase not only the occurrence but also the mortality rate of colonic cancer (Trowell 1976). The presence of fiber in the diet is also thought to act as a protective agent against other noninfectious diseases. For example, dietary fiber's relationship to congestive heart disease has been investigated (Trowell 1972). Increased levels of dietary fiber may promote the reduction of blood cholesterol levels (Trowell 1976; Balmer and Zilversmit 1974). There may even be a relationship between dietary fiber intake and atherosclerosis. Much more investigative work needs to take place to clarify any relationships that may exist between dietary fiber intake and blood cholesterol levels and also the presence or absence of other disease states such as colitis, diverticulosis, appendicitis, and hemorrhoids.

Fiber and Stress

Several stress-related disorders associated with disturbances of the gastrointestinal tract may be either directly or indirectly influenced by the presence of fiber in the diet. Although the role of fiber in the diet does not appear to play a direct role in the elicitation of the stress response, it may perhaps be altered in its activity and effectiveness as reflected by stress induced changes in the gastroentestinal system. Further research is needed to clarify the relationship of dietary fiber, if any, to various types of stress exposures.

GARLIC

Garlic contains large amounts of vitamin B and C and calcium, phosphorus, and potassium. Many Europeans and Russians have long considered it to have medicinal properties. Claims have been made for its role in reducing high blood pressure and reducing excess amounts of sugar. While much more research is needed to clarify its role, garlic may be an effective adjunct to the diet in ameliorating many stress-related disorders.

GINSENG

Although ginseng is not categorized in Western culture as a necessary nutrient, it has been used in the Orient for almost 2,000 years as a general tonic and as a tonic for retarding the process of aging. It is also used as an energy booster and is used medicinally by Chinese physicians to treat weakness and fatigue. Even though ginseng is not considered to be a nutrient and has not been used in the West, some researchers have described a possible influence of ginseng in the stress response.

The pharmacological action of ginseng has not been very well investigated, but some evidence indicates that the drug may affect the different body systems, including the digestive system (Yoon 1960) and the cardiovascular system (Wood et al. 1964).

Ginseng and Stress

Some researchers report that the administration of ginseng extracts to animals exposed to cold (Kim 1963) and acceleration stress (Kim 1966) significantly reduced their mortality rate. Kim et al. (1970) report further experiments that demonstrate the influence of ginseng on the stress mechanism. They demonstrate that in laboratory rats subjected to either cold or heat stress, the initial stress-induced depletion of ascorbic acid content of the adrenal glands was followed by a restoration. The adrenal ascorbic acid recovery process was significantly facilitated by ginseng administration. In another experiment, these researchers report that even without the presence of the pituitary gland (total hypophysectomy), ginseng still facilitated both the depletion and subsequent restoration of the ascorbic acid content of the adrenal gland in response to ACTH. They conclude that ginseng may exert its action upon a peripheral site of the stress mechanism as opposed to a more central site as a result of the elicitation of the stress response. Needless to say, much more investigative work needs to be done to clarify the role of this drug both in its medicinal role and in its role in the stress mechanism of the body.

KELP

There are several forms of kelp. The seaweed form is the most common and is a very rich source of many vitamins and several minerals. In addition, kelp contains several of the trace minerals. Because of its iodine content, it is thought to be beneficial for the thyroid gland. Kelp also promotes healthy mucous membranes. It has been reported that kelp has beneficial effects in counteracting nervous system disorders, constipation, and skin irritations. In view of its vitamin and mineral content, kelp may prove to be an effective food supplement in times of stress.

LECITHIN

Lecithin forms an integral part of every cell in the body. Its importance lies in its ability to break down cholesterol and permit its passage through blood vessels. It therefore may play a role in the prevention of atherosclerosis. Lecithin is found in the myelin sheath of nerves and therefore helps to maintain the integrity of the nervous system. It is also thought to aid in a cleansing action of the kidneys and the liver.

ROSE HIPS

Rose hips are the seeds found at the base of the rose. They are a rich source of vitamin C. Rose hips are generally used together with vitamin C supplements.

SPIRULINA

Spirulina which is a microscopic blue-green algae is a high-protein food. It is approximately 65 percent protein and is therefore the highest known protein source. The protein in spirulina contains all the eight essential amino acids, and therefore it is a complete protein. It contains vitamins A, E, H, and K, and all of the B complex vitamins, containing the highest natural source of vitamin B_{12}. Spirulina is also rich in magnesium, potassium, phosphorus, and all of the necessary trace elements, cell salts, and digestive enzymes. It contains high levels of chlorophyll, ferrodoxins, and other pigments. Because of its ingredients, spirulina is considered by many researchers to be a whole nutritious compact survival food. It may be an appropriate supplementary or additive food in times of stress.

WHEAT GERM

Wheat germ is the kernel part of wheat. It is rich in protein, the B complex vitamins, vitamin E, and several important minerals. Because of its high nutrient value, wheat germ may prove to be a very beneficial food supplement in times of stress.

YEAST

Yeast is a very rich source of iron and the B complex vitamins. It is also an excellent source of protein. Yeast contains several minerals and amino acids. Because of its nutritional content, it may be beneficial in supplying needed nutrients in times of stress.

10

SUMMARY

The living organism, under normal conditions, is maintained in a state of physiological homeostasis. This state is regulated and characterized by physiological processes involving metabolism and operating in a precise dynamic balance. The underlying biochemistry involves a complex interaction of many of the vitamins, minerals, enzymes, hormones, etc., including several interrelationships among them. This text has described many of the nutrients that are considered essential for human health. These nutrients are listed in Table 10.1. When, however, conditions and circumstances affecting the organism change, such as through stress, several regulatory mechanisms come into play to regain and maintain physiological homeostasis. Many of the regulatory mechanisms that influence the metabolic changes that take place in the body involve the interaction between a neural axis, a neuroendocrine axis, and metabolism.

The elicitation of the stress response results in an increase in the metabolic needs of the body. This increase in metabolism is an attempt by the body to maintain homeostasis. To meet the increased metabolic needs, the adrenal gland secretes its hormones into the circulation. These hormones prepare the body to take action, to fight or take flight from the stressful event. These adrenal hormones as well as several other stress hormones accelerate many of the physiological processes in the body. For example, heart rate and blood pressure increase, muscle tension increases, and breathing patterns change. Stress hormones aid in the acceleration of protein, carbohydrate, and fat metabolism. This elevated metabolism provides the body with extra stores of energy as well as instant energy, which it can use in times of emergency and stress.

TABLE 10.1 Nutrients Considered Essential for Human Health that Must be Obtained from Food Sources

	Water
	Carbohydrates
	Fats
	Proteins
Amino Acids:	Isoleucine, Leucine, Lysine, Methionine, Phenylalanine, Threonine, Tryptophan, Valine, Arginine, Histidine (needed for growth in children)
Vitamins:	Vitamins A, C, D, E, K, B_1, B_2, B_5, B_6, B_{12}, Niacin, Folic Acid, Biotin
Minerals:	Calcium, Chlorine, Chromium, Cobalt, Copper, Iodine, Iron, Magnesium, Manganese, Molybdenum, Phosphorus, Potassium, Selenium, Sodium, Sulfur, Zinc

As a result of the increased metabolism, there is an increase in the use and excretion of many nutrients, including some of the minerals. Some of the vitamins may also be used and become deficient in the body as a result of acute or chronic stress. A good example is the stress-induced decrease in the body's stores of vitamin C. During conditions of stress, vitamin C is used by the adrenal gland. Should the stress response become chronic, or should the stressful event be experienced as severe or intense, a depletion of vitamin C may occur in the adrenal gland and in other body tissues.

Nutrient changes that take place in the body as a result of the stress response have been described in the text. The experience of acute stress may not lead to any major loss or depletion of any of the nutrients. The more intense the stress experienced, however, the greater the use of these nutrients and the more likely that some may be lost from the body. Chronic stress is more likely to decrease the nutrient stores.

Besides the stress-induced changes that occur in the vitamins and minerals, the stress-induced changes in the metabolism of proteins, carbohydrates, and fats were also described in the text. In particular, for greater energy production, carbohydrate and fat use increases as a result of the elicitation of the stress response. Depending on the intensity and chronicity of the stress, an increase in protein metabolism leading to a negative nitrogen balance may also occur. A summary of these changes is shown in Tables 10.2 and 10.3.

In view of the information provided, the nutrients, including the vitamins and minerals that may prove to be beneficial during times of stress, should include those listed in Table 10.4. The B complex vitamins

TABLE 10.2. Changes in Proteins, Carbohydrates, Fats, and Other Metabolites as a Result of Stress

---

Increase in the use of

    Carbohydrates → increase in blood sugar
    Fats   → increase in free fatty acids
    Proteins   → negative nitrogen balance (under more intense and
                      chronic stress)

Increase in

    Enzyme production and activity
    Water retention

Increase or Decrease in

    Plasma uric acid levels

---

and vitamin C are rapidly used by the body and could become depleted in times of stress, particularly chronic stress. If vitamin supplementation is chosen during such times of stress, it should at the very least include the vitamin B complex family and vitamin C. In addition, calcium, magnesium, phosphorus, and potassium would be among the important minerals that should be included as part of a vitamin mineral supplement.

There are several disorders and disease states that are associated with the experience of stress. However, some of these disorders may not so much be a direct result of the elicitation of the stress response itself but may be more directly related to the nutrient imbalance or deficiencies that may occur as a result of the experience of stress.

Therefore, it is important that individuals who experience the stress response, particularly if it is chronic, work toward the achievement and maintenance of a well-balanced diet. This diet should encompass all of the nutrients, vitamins, minerals, proteins, carbohydrates, and fats, with particular emphasis on replacing nutrients that have been lost or become deficient.

In view of the emphasis of this text, it seems appropriate to recall what Hippocrates said approximately 2,500 years ago. He said, "Our food must be our medicine—our medicine must be our food." Also, it seems appropriate to close with a quote by Thomas Alva Edison. "The doctor of the future will prescribe no drugs, but will interest his patients in the care and nutrition of the human frame and in the cause and prevention of disease."

TABLE 10.3. Vitamins and Minerals that are Altered as a Result of Stress

DECREASE

Vitamins: A, C, D, E, K, B complex, B_1, B_2, B_5, B_6, B_{12}, niacin, folic acid

Minerals: Calcium, chromium, iron, magnesium, phosphorus, potassium, zinc

INCREASE

Minerals: Sodium, chloride, copper

TABLE 10.4. Nutrient that may be Beneficial During Times of Stress

Nutrients

Carbohydrates, fats, proteins

Vitamins

Vitamin A, C, D, E, K
Vitamin B complex, including B_1, B_2, B_5, B_6, B_{12}, folic acid, niacin, biotin, choline, inositol, PABA

Minerals

Calcium, chromium, iron, magnesium, phosphorus, potassium, zinc

APPENDIX

TABLE A-1. Sources and RDA of Vitamins

Vitamin	Sources	U.S. Recommended Daily Allowance (RDA) Adults and Children 4 Years and Over
A (Retinol)	dairy products, eggs, fish and fish liver oils. (Good sources of carotene, from which the body makes its own vitamin A are colored fruits and vegetables)	5,000 IU
B_1 (Thiamin)	brewer's yeast, brown rice, fish, organ meats, pork, poultry, whole wheat, wheat germ, oatmeal, peanuts, most vegetables, milk, soybeans, peas, lentils, dried beans	1.5 mg
B_2 (Riboflavin)	brewer's yeast, milk, nuts, whole grains, organ meats, cheese, fish, eggs	1.7 mg
B_5 (Pantothenic acid)	yeast, organ meats, wheat, wheat germ, salmon, whole grains	5–10 mg
B_6 (Pyridoxine)	brewer's yeast, meat, organ meats, fish, egg yolk, beets, most leafy vegetables, milk, yeast, wheat germ, whole grains, blackstrap molasses	2.0 mg
B_{12} (Cyanocobalamin)	eggs, milk, milk products, cheese, organ meats, pork, most meats	6 µg
B_{15} (Pangamic acid)	whole grains, brewer's yeast, brown meat, organ meats, seeds (sunflower, sesame, pumpkin)	—
Niacin (Niacinamide)	whole wheat products, yeast, lean meats, green vegetables, eggs, nuts, legumes	20 mg
Biotin	whole grains, organ meats, yeast, legumes, milk, egg yolk	0.3 mg

Vitamin	Sources	U.S. Recommended Daily Allowance (RDA) Adults and Children 4 Years and Over
Folic Acid (Folacin)	organ meats, yeast, deep green leafy vegetables, whole grains, milk, milk products, salmon	0.4 mg
Choline	egg yolks, green leafy vegetables, legumes, fish, wheat germ, soybeans, lecithin	—
Inositol	citrus fruits, brewer's yeast, nuts, milk, meat, whole grains, vegetables, lecithin, corn, oatmeal	—
PABA (*para*-aminobenzoic acid)	brewer's yeast, whole grains, organ meats, wheat germ, blackstrap molasses	—
Vitamin C (ascorbic acid)	citrus fruits, green peppers, berries, cantaloupe, greens, cabbage	60 mg
Vitamin D	sunshine, fish liver oils, bone meal, eggs, milk, butter, fat, organ meats	400 IU
Vitamin E (Tocopherol)	eggs, organ meats, wheat germ, vegetable oils, green leafy vegetables, whole grain cereals	10–15 IU
Vitamin F (unsaturated fatty acids)	vegetable oils such as cottonseed, peanut, safflower, corn, and linseed	—
Vitamin H (See Biotin)		
Vitamin K	green vegetables, alfalfa, egg yolk, soybean oil (synthesized by bacteria in the intestine)	—
Vitamin P (Bioflavinoids)	pulp of citrus fruits, rose hips, apricots, asparagus	—
Rutin (Included in Vitamin P)	buckwheat, rose hips	—

Note: g = gram; mg = milligram; μg = microgram; IU = International Unit (an International Unit is approximately equal to one milligram); 1,000 μg = 1 mg; 1,000 mg = 1 g.

TABLE A-II. Sources and RDA of Minerals

Mineral	Sources	RDA
Calcium	molasses, yogurt, bone meal, milk, cheese, fresh green leafy vegetables, oily fish	1.0 g
Chromium	brewer's yeast, corn oil, whole grain cereals and breads, shellfish, blackstrap molasses, mushrooms, beer, grape juice	—
Cobalt	vitamin B_{12}, meat, fish, eggs, dairy products	—
Copper	blackstrap molasses, nuts, organ meats, seafood, raisins, bone meal, malted products, cocoa	2 mg
Iodine	seafood, kelp, peanuts, fish liver oil, iodized salt	150 µg
Iron	blackstrap mollases, eggs, fish, organ meats, beef, poultry, wheat germ, dried apricots, soybeans, sardines, dark green vegetables	18 mg
Magnesium	green vegetables, bran, honey, seafood, bone meal, seeds, nuts, beans, spinach, kelp, soybeans	400 mg
Manganese	bran, cereals, egg yolks, whole grains, dark leafy vegetables, legumes, nuts, pineapples, bananas	—
Phosphorus	eggs, fish, cheese, meat, poultry, grains	1.0 g
Potassium	blackstrap molasses, raisins, apricots (dried), nuts, whole grains, seafood, wheat germ, greens, tomato juice, figs, unpeeled potatoes, dried fruits, soy flour	—
Selenium	seafood, meats	50–200 µg
Silicon	beer, unrefined cereals	—
Sodium	salt, milk, cheese, seafood, almost all prepared foods, bread, butter, bacon, margarine, corned and pickled meat, sausages, breakfast cereals	—
Sulfur	bran, cheese, eggs, nuts, wheat germ, fish, protein foods	—

TABLE A-II. Sources and RDA of Minerals *(continued)*

Mineral	*Sources*	*RDA*
Vanadium	root vegetables, nuts, unrefined cereals	—
Zinc	brewer's yeast, soybeans, seafood, mushrooms, meat, whole grains, spinach, sunflower seeds, nuts	15 mg

Note: g = gram; mg = milligram; μg = microgram; 1,000 μg = 1 mg; 1,000 mg = 1 g.
To compare the above amounts it is helpful to note that one level teaspoon of white sugar weighs approximately 4 g. .

BIBLIOGRAPHY

CHAPTER 1

Asterita, M.F. 1985. *The Physiology of Stress: With Special Reference to the Neuroendocrine System*. New York: Human Sciences Press.

Everly, G. Jr., and F. Rosenfeld. 1981. *The Nature and Treatment of the Stress Response*. New York: Plenum Press.

Selye, H. 1976. *Stress in Health and Disease*. Reading, Mass.: Butterworths.

_____. 1957. *The Stress of Life*. London: Longmans, Green.

_____. 1950. *The Physiology and Pathology of Exposure to Stress*. Montreal: Acta Inc. Medical Publishers.

CHAPTER 2

Galbo, H., J.J. Holst, and N.J. Christensen. 1975. "Glucagon and Plasma Catecholamine Response to Graded and Prolonged Exercise in Man." *Journal of Applied Physiology* 38: 90.

Heath, G.W., A.A. Ehsani, J.M. Hagberg, J.M. Henderleter, and A.P. Goldbert. 1983. "Exercise Training Improves Lipoprotein Lipid Profiles in Patients with Coronary Artery Disease." *American Heart Journal* 105: 889.

Kibler, R.F., W.J. Taylor, and J.D. Mvers. 1984. "Effect of Glucagon on Net Splanchnic Balance of Glucose, Amino Acid, Nitrogen Urea, Ketone and Oxygen in Man." *Journal of Clinical Investigation* 43, 904.

Le Blanc, J., A. Nadeau, M. Boulay, and S. Rousseau-Migneron. 1979. "Effects of Physical Training and Adiposity on Glucose Metabolism and ^{125} I-insulin Binding." *Journal of Applied Physiology* 46: 235.

Lohman, D., F. Liebold, W. Heilman, H. Senger, and A. Pohl. 1978. "Diminished Insulin Response to Highly Trained Athletes." *Metabolism* 27: 521.

Mondon, C.E., C.B. Dolkes, and G. Reaven. 1980. "Site of Enhanced Insulin Activity in Exercise-trained Rats at Rest." *American Journal of Physiology* 239: E169.

Richard, D., A. Labrie, D. Lupien, A. Tremblay, and J. LeBlanc. 1982. "Interactions Between Dietary Obesity and Exercise Training on Carbohydrate Metabolism." *International Journal of Obesity* 6: 359.

Roth, J., and C. Grunfeld. 1981. "Endocrine Systems: Mechanisms of Disease, Target Cells and Receptors. In *Textbook of Endocrinology* edited by R.H. Williams. Philadelphia: Saunders.

Sutton, J.R. 1983. "The Hormonal Responses to Exercise at Sea Level and at altitude." In *Hypoxia, Exercise and Altitude: Proceedings of the Third Banff International Hypoxia Symposium*. New York: Alan R. Liss.

———. 1978."Hormonal and Metabolic Responses to Exercise in Subjects of High and Low Work Capacities." *Medical Science Sports* 10: 1.

Vranic, M., and M. Berger. 1979. "Exercise and Diabetes Mellitus." *Diabetes* 28: 147.

CHAPTER 3

Arroyane, G., D. Wilson, J. Mendez, M. Behar, and N.S. Scrimshaw, 1961. "Serum and Liver Vitamin A and Lipids in Children with Severe Protein Malnutrition." *American Journal of Clinical Nutrition* 9: 180.

Barisov, I.F. 1977. "Retinol Requirement of Students Engaged in Sports." *Teoriia I Praktika Fizicheskoi Kultury*, p. 58.

Bender, H.J., D.C. Herting, V. Hurst, S.C. Finch, and H.M. Spiro. 1965 "Tocopheral Deficiency in Man." *New England Journal of Medicine* 273: 1289.

Calvert, C.C., M.C. Nesheim, and M.L. Scott. 1962. "Effectiveness of Selenium on the Prevention of Nutritional Muscular Dystrophy in the Chick." *Proceedings of the Society of Experimental Biology and Medicine* 109: 16.

Charles, O.W., and E.J. Day. 1968. "The Response of Vitamin K Deficient Chicks Subjected to Heat Stress." *Poultry Sciences* 47: 1996.

Chernov, M.S., F.B. Cook, B.S. McDonald Wood, and H.W. Hale. 1969. "Stress Ulcer: A Preventable Disease." *Journal of Trauma* 12: 831.

Chernov, M.S., H.W. Hale Jr., and B.S. McDonald Wood. 1971 "Prevention of Stress Ulcers." *American Journal of Surgery* 122: 674.

Committee on Diet, Nutrition and Cancer. 1982. *Diet, Nutrition and Cancer*. Washington, D.C.: National Academy Press.

Cordes, D.V., and A.H. Mosher. 1966. "Brown Pigmentation (Lipo-fuscinosis) of the Canine Intestinal Muscularis." *Journal of Pathology and Bacteriology* 92: 197.

Denyes, A., and J.D. Carter. 1961. "Clotting Time of Cold Exposed and Hibernating Hamsters." *Nature* 190: 450.

Deshmukh, D.S., P. Malathi, and J. Ganguly. 1964. "Studies on Metabolism of Vitamin A. 5. Dietary Protein and Metabolism of Vitamin A." *Biochemical Journal* 90: 98.

Diplock, A.T., J. Green, J. Bunyan, D. McHale, and I.R. Muthy. 1967. "Vitamin E and Stress. 3. The Metabolism of d-alpha-Tocopherol in the Rat under Dietary Stress with Silver." *British Journal of Nutrition* 21: 115.

Dougherty, T.F., and A. White. 1945. "Functional Alterations in Lymphoid Tissue Induced by Adrenal Cortical Secretion." *American Journal of Anatomy* 77: 81.

Eriksson F., S.V. Johansson, H. Mellsledt, O. Strandberg, and P.O. Wester. 1974. "Iron Intoxication in Two Adult Patients." *Acta Medica Scandanavica* 196: 231.

Evans, H.M., and K.S. Bishop. 1923. "Existence of a Hitherto Unknown Dietary Factor Essential for Reproduction." *Journal of the American Medical Association* 81: 889.

Evensen, S.A., R. Forde, I. Opedal, and H. Stormorken. 1982. "Acute Iron Intoxication with Abruptly Reduced Levels of Vitamin K-dependent Coagulation Factors." *Scandanavian Journal of Haemotology* 29: 25.

Felix, E.L., B. Loyd, and M.H. Cohen. 1975. "Inhibition of the Growth and Development of a Transplantable Murine Melanoma by Vitamin A." *Science* 189: 886.

Food and Nutrition Board 1980. *Recommended Dietary Allowances*, 9th ed. Washington D.C.: National Academy of Sciences, National Research Council.

Glick, D., P.K. Nakane, S. Levine, and L. Jones. 1966. "Influence of ACTH, Food Restriction and Electric Shock on Total Vitamin A in the Rat Adrenal Gland and on its Quantitative Histological Distribution." *Endocrinology* 78: 945.

Green, J., and J. Bunyan. 1969. "Vitamin E and the Biological Antioxidant Theory." *Nutrition Abstracts and Reviews* 39: 321.

Green, J., A.T. Diplock, J. Bunyan, D. McHale, and I.R. Muthy, 1967a. "Vitamin E and Stress. 1. Dietary Unsaturated Fatty Acid Stress and the Metabolism of alpha-Tocopherol in the rat." *British Journal of Nutrition* 21: 169.

Green, J., I.R. Muthy, A.T. Diplock, J. Bunyan, M.A. Cawthorne, and E.A. Murrell. 1976b. "Vitamin E and Stress: The Interrelationships Between Polyunsaturated Fatty Acid Stress, Vitamin A and Vitamin E in the Rat and the Chick." *British Journal of Nutrition* 21: 845.

Harris, P.L., and K.E. Mason. 1956. *Proceedings of the Third International Congress on Vitamin E.* Venice.

Hayes, K.C., S.W. Nielsen, and J.E. Rousseau Jr. 1969. "Vitamin E Deficiency and Fat Stress in the Dog." *Journal of Nutrition* 99: 196.

Henriksson P., L. Nilsson, I.M. Nilsson, and P. Stenberg. 1979. "Fatal Iron Intoxication with Multiple Coagulation Defects and Degradation of Factor VIII and Factor XIII. *Scandanavian Journal of Haemotology* 22: 235.

Hepner, R., and N.C. Maiden. 1971. "Growth Rate, Nutrient Intake and 'mothering'; As Determinants of Malnutrition in Disadvantaged Children." *Nutrition Reviews* 29: 219.

Horwitt, M.K. 1980. "Therapeutic Uses of Vitamin E in Medicine." *Nutrition Reviews* 38: 105.

_____. 1962. "Interrelations Between Vitamin E and Polunsaturated Fatty Acids in Adult Men." *Vitamins Hormones* 20: 541.

Jamieson, D. and H.A.S. van den Brenk. 1964. "Effects of Antioxidants on High Pressure Oxygen Toxicity." *Biochemical Pharmacology* 13: 159.

Kark, J.D., A.H. Smith, B.R. Switzer and C.G. Hames. 1981. "Serum Vitamin A (Retinol) and Cancer Incidence in Evans County, Georgia." *Journal of the National Cancer Institute* 66: 7.

Kasper, H., M. Brodersen, and R. Schedel. 1975. "Concentration of Vitamin A, Retinol-binding Protein and Prealbumin in Serum in Response to Stress. A Contribution to the Prevention of Stress Ulcers by Means of Vitamin A." *Acta Hepato-Gastroenterologica* 22: 403.

Kinley, L.J., and R.F. Krause. 1959. "Influence of Vitamin A on Cholesterol Blood Levels." *Proceedings of the Society of Experimental Biology* 102: 353.

Krause, R.F., M.A. Pallotta, and I.I. Yoder. 1968. "Lipid Alterations in Beagles Produced by Atherogenic Stress and Vitamin A." *Journal of Atherosclerosis Research* 8: 277.

Martin, M.S., R. Lambert, F. Martin, and C. Andre. 1967. "Effet Protecteur de la Vitamine A sur l'Ulcère de Contrainte du Rat. *Comptes Rendus des Séances de la Société de Biologie et de ses Fidiales* (Paris) 161: 2527.

McCollum, E.V. 1957. *A History of Nutrition.* Boston: Houghton Mifflin.

McCormick, D.L., F.J. Burns, and R.E. Albert. 1981. "Inhibition of Benzo [alpha] Pyrene Induced Mammary Carcinogenesis by Retinyl Acetate." *Journal of the National Cancer Institute* 66: 559.

Mills, C.A., E. Cottingham, and M. Mills. 1944. "Environmental Temperature and Vitamin K Deficiency. *American Journal of Physiology* 141: 359.

Moacelli, R., and V. Pala. 1969. "Influenza della Vitamin A sull Ulcers Gastrica Experimentall del Ratto. *Pathologica* 61: 387.

Moore, T. 1940. "The Effect of Vitamin E Deficiency on the Vitamin A Reserves in the Rat." *Biochemical Journal* 34: 1321.

Morita, A., and K. Nakano. 1982. "Effect of Chronic Immobilization Stress on Tissue Distribution of Vitamin A in Rats Fed a Diet with Adequate Vitamin A." *American Journal of Nutrition* 112: 789.

Nakano, K., and A. Morita. 1982. "Redistribution of Vitamin A in Tissues of Rats with Imposed Chronic Confinement Stress." *British Journal of Nutrition* 47: 645.

Page, H.M., E.S. Erwin, and G.E. Nelms. 1959. "Effect of Heat and Solar Radiation on Vitamin A Utilization by the Bovine Animal." *American Journal of Physiology* 196:917.

Porter, E., and E.J. Masoro. 1961. "Effect of Cold Acclimation on Vitamin A Metabolism." *Proceedings of the Society for Experimental Biology and Medicine* 108: 609.

Ramsden, D.B., H.P. Price, W.A. Burr, A.R. Bradwell, E.G. Block, A.E. Evance, and H. Hoffenberg. 1978. "The Interrelationship of Thyroid Hormones, Vitamin A and Other Binding Proteins Following Acute Stress." *Clinical Endocrinology* 8: 109.

Rechcegl, M., Jr., S. Berger, J.K. Loosli, and H.H. Williams. 1962. "Dietary Protein and the Utilization of Vitamin A." *Journal of Nutrition* 76: 435.

Reddy, V. 1981. "Fat Soluble Vitamin Deficiencies in Children in Relation to Protein Energy Malnutrition and Environmental Stress." In *Nutrition in Health and Disease and International Development: Symposia from the XII International Congress of Nutrition.* New York: Alan R. Liss.

Reddy, V., and S.G. Srikantia. 1966. "Serum Vitamin A in Kwashiorkor." *American Journal of Clinical Nutrition* 18: 105.

Reich, C. 1975. "Allergy and Diseases of the Central Nervous System." *Journal of Orthomolecular Psychiatry* 4: 269.

Rettura, G., A. Schitlek, M. Hardy, S.M. Levenson, A. Demetriou, and E. Seifter. 1975. "Antitumor Action of Vitamin A in Mice Inoculated with Adenocarcinoma cells." *Journal of the National Cancer Institute* 54: 1489.

Riley, V. 1975. "Mouse Mammary Tumors: Alteration of Incidence as Apparent Function of Stress." *Science* 189: 465.

Rubenstein, E., and A. Lack. 1960. "Extremity Venous Blood Temperature and Blood Clotting Mechanisms." *Journal of Applied Physiology* 15: 598.

Santisteban, G.A. 1953. Abstracts. *Anatomical Record* 115: 226.

Santisteban, G., and T.F. Dougherty. 1954. "Comparison of the Influence of Adrenocortical Hormones on the Growth and Involution of Lymphatic Organs." *Endocrinology* 54: 130.

Schwartz, K. 1965. "Role of Vitamin E, Selenium, and Related Factors in Experimental Nutritional Liver Disease." *Federation Proceedings* 24: 58.

Seifter, E. 1976. Of Stress, Vitamin A and Tumors. *Science* 193: 74.

Seifter, E., G. Rettura, M. Zisblatt, S.M. Levenson, N. Levine, A. Davidson, and J. Seifter. 1973a. "Enhancement of Tumor Development in Physically Stressed Mice Inoculated with an Oncogenic Virus." *Experientia* 29: 1379.

Seifter, E., M. Zisblatt, N. Levine, and G. Rettura. 1973b. "Inhibitory Action of Vitamin A on a Murine Sarcoma." *Life Sciences* 13: 945.

Seifter, E., M. Zisblatt, and G. Rettura. 1973c. Abstract 42. In 166th National Meeting of the American Chemical Society.

Selye, H. 1956. *The Stress of Life.* New York: McGraw Hill.

Sen, I.P. 1965. "Effect of Different Fats on Some Biochemical Values in Rats with Vitamin E Deficiency." *Nutrition Abstracts and Reviews* 35: 2037.

Sporn, M.B., N.M. Dunlop, D.L. Newton, and J.M. Smith. 1976. "Prevention of Chemical Carcinogenesis by Vitamin A and Its Synthetic Analogs (Retinoids)." *Federation Proceedings* 35: 1332.

Sundaresan, P.R., and G.H. Sundaresan. 1975. "Tissue Distribution of Retinol and Its Metabolites after Administration of Double-labelled Retinol." *Biochemical Journal* 152: 99.

Sundaresan, P.R., V.G. Winters, and D.G. Therreault. 1967. "Effect of Low Environmental Temperature on the Metabolism of Vitamin A." *Journal of Nutrition* 92: 474.

Surekha Rao, M.S., K. Thyagarajan, G.S. Kishore, and H.R. Cama 1974. "Vitamin A Metabolism under Nutritional Stress." *International Journal for Vitamin and Nutrition Research* 44: 151.

Taylor, D.W. 1953. *Journal of Physiology* Abstract 121.

Toffler, A.H., R.B. Hurkill and H.M. Spiro. 1963. "Brown Bowel Syndrome." *Annals of Internal Medicine* 58, 872.

Van Vleet, J.F., A.H. Rebar, and V.J. Ferrans. 1977. "Acute Cobalt and Isoproterenol Cardiotoxicity in Swine: Protection by Selenium–Vitamin E Supplementation and Potentiation by Stress-susceptible Phenotype. *American Journal of Veterinary Research* 38: 991.

Wald, N., M. Idle, J. Boreham, and A. Bailey. 1980. "Low Serum–Vitamin A and Subsequent Risk of Cancer: Preliminary Results of a Prospective Study." *Lancet* 2: 813.

Willett, W.C., B.F. Polk, B.A. Underwood, M.J. Stampfer, S. Pressel, B. Rosner, J.O. Taylor, K. Schneider, and C.G. Hames. 1984. "Relation of Serum Vitamins A and E and Carotenoids to the Risk of Cancer." *New England Journal of Medicine* 310: 430.

Wilson, S.J., H.E. Heath, P.L. Nulson, and G.G. Ens. 1958. "Blood Coagulation in Acute Iron Intoxication." *Blood* 13: 483.

Wood, J.D., and J. Topliff. 1961. "The Comparative Hypocholesterolemic Activities of Fish Oil and Vitamin A." *Journal of the Fisheries Research Board of Canada* 18: 377.

Zisblatt, M., M. Hardy, G. Rettura, E. Seifter. 1973. "Partial Inhibition of a Murine Sarcoma by Vitamin A." Abstract 30 *Journal of Nutrition* 103.

CHAPTER 4

Altschul, R., ed. 1965. *Niacin in Vascular Disorders and Hyperlipemia.* Springfield, Ill. Charles C. Thomas.

Anderson, T.W. 1975. "Large-scale Trials of Vitamin C." *Annals of the New York Academy of Sciences* 258: 498.

Barker, H., and O. Frank. 1968. "Vitamin Status in Metabolic Upsets." *World Review of Nutrition and Dietetics* 6: 124. (Basel, New York: Karger.)

Ben Nathan, D., E.D. Heller, and M. Perek 1976. "The Effect of Short Heat Stress upon Leucocyte Count, Plasma Corticosterone Level, Plasma and Leucocyte Ascorbic Acid Content." *British Poultry Science* 17:481.

Benes, V., and V. Hrubes. 1968. "Serum Free Fatty Acids Level after an Experimentally Induced Emotional Stress and Its Modification by Nicotinic Acid in Rats with Different Charcteristics of Higher Nervous Activity." *Activitas Nervosa Superior (Praha)* 10: 395.

Bombelli, R., T. Farkas, and R. Vertua. 1965. "Investigation on the Effect of Nicotinic Acid on Plasma Free Fatty Acid Levels." *Medicina et Pharmacologia Experimentatis* 12: 8.

Brook, M., and J.J. Gremshaw. 1968. "Vitamin C Concentration of Plasma and Leukocytes as Related to Smoking Habit, Age, and Sex of Humans." *American Journal of Clinical Nutrition* 21: 1254.

Carlson, L.A. 1965. "Inhibition of the Mobilization of Free Fatty Acids from Adipose Tissue." *Annals of the New York Academy of Sciences* 131: 119.

_____. 1963. "Studies on the Effect of Nicotinic Acid on Catecholamine Stimulated Lipolysis in Adipose Tissue in Vitro." *Acta Medica Scandinavica* 173: 719.

Carlson, L.A., J. Boberg, and B. Hogstedt 1965. "Some Physiological and Clinical Implications of Lipid Mobilization from Adipose Tissue." In *Handbook of Physiology. V. Adipose Tissue.* edited by A.E. Renold and G.F. Cahill, p. 625. Washington, D.C.: American Physiological Society.

Carlson, L.A., R.J. Havel, L.G. Eke'und, and A. Holmgre. 1963. "Effect of Nicotinic Acid on the Turnover Rate and Oxidation of the Free Fatty Acids of Plasma in Man during Exercise." *Metabolism* 12: 837.

Carlson, L.A., L. Levi, and L. Orö. 1968. "Plasma Lipids and Urinary Excretion of Cathecholamines in Man during Experimentally Induced Emotional Stress and Their Modification by Nicotinic Acid." *Journal of Clinical Investigation* 47: 1795.

Carlson, L.A., and L. Orö. 1962. "The Effect of Nicotinic Acid on the Plasma Free Fatty Acids." *Acta Medica Scandinavica* 172: 641.

Carlson, L.A., and B. Pernow. 1959. "Studies on Blood Lipids during Exercise." *Journal of Laboratory and Clinical Medicine* 53: 833.

Cheney, C.D., and E. Rudrud. 1974. "Prophylaxis by Vitamin C in Starvation Induced Rat Stomach Ulceration." *Life Sciences* 14: 2209.

Civen, M., J.E. Leeb, R.M. Wishnow, and R.J. Morin 1980. "Effects of Dietary Ascorbic Acid and Vitamin E Deficiency on Rat Adrenal Cholesterol Ester Metabolism and Corticosteroid Genesis." *International Journal of Vitamin Nutrition Research* 50: 70.

Dettman, G. "Vitamin C—Latest Development." 1973. *Journal of the Australasian College of Biomedical Scientists* p. 609.

Dettman, G., and I. Zimmerman, 1973. "A Report of Australian League Footballers Supplemented with Vitamin C." *Journal of the Australasian College of Biomedical Scientists* p. 50.

Elwood, P.C., R.E. Hughes and R.J. Hurley. 1970. "Ascorbic Acid and Serum-Cholesterol." *Lancet* 2: 1197.

Evans, J.R., R.E. Hughes, and P.R. Jones. 1967. *Proceedings of the Nutrition Society* 27: 36.

Glavin, G.B., W.P. Paré, and G.P. Vicent, Jr. 1978. "Ascorbic Acid and Stress Ulcer in the Rat." *Journal of Nutrition* 108: 1969.

Goldstein, J.L., J.J. Albers, W.R. Hazzard, H.R. Schrott, E.L. Bierman, and A.G. Motulsky. 1973. "Genetic and Medical Significance of Neonatal Hyper-lipidemia." *Journal of Clinical Investigation* 52: 1523.

Gross, R.L., J.V.O. Reid, P.M. Newberne, B. Burgess, C. Marston, and W. Hift. 1975. "Depressed Cell-mediated Immunity in Megaloblastic Anemia due to Folic Acid Deficiency." *American Journal of Clinical Nutrition* 28: 225.

Heindel, J.J., and T.R. Riggs. 1978. "Amino Acid Transport in Vitamin B_6 Deficient Rats: Dependence on Growth Hormone Supply." *American Journal of Physiology* 235: E316.

Henschel, A.H., et al. 1944. "Vitamin C and Ability to Work in Hot Environments." *American Journal of Tropical Medicine* 24: 259.

Hodges, R.E. 1970. "The Effects of Stress on Ascorbic Acid Metabolism in Man." *Nutrition* 5: 11.

Hoffer, A. 1963. "Nicotinic Acid: An Adjunct in the Treatment of Schizophrenia." *American Journal of Psychiatry* 120: 171.

Hrubes, V., and V. Benes. 1967. "The Plasma Level of Non-esterified Fatty an Indicator of Stress." *Activitas Nervosa Superior (Praha)* 9: 241.

Hughes, R.E., and P. Nicholas 1971. "Effects of Caging on the Ascorbic Acid Content of the Adrenal Glands of the Guinea-pig and Gerbil." *Life Sciences* 10: 53.

Irwin, E., A.R. Buchanan, B.B. Longwell, O. Holtkamp, and R.M. Hill. 1950. "Ascorbic Acid Content of Adrenal Glands of Young Albino Rats after Cold and Other Stresses." *Endocrinology* 46: 526.

Kahlson, G., and E. Rosengren. 1968. "New Approaches to the Physiology of Histamine." *Physiological Reviews* 48: 155.

Kamala, S., R. Jaya, and P.S. Mohan. 1982. "Plasma Somatomedin Activity, Growth Hormone and Insulin Levels in Vitamin B_6 Deficient Rats." *Hormone and Metabolic Research* 14: 580.

Kotzé, J.P. 1975. "The Effects of Vitamin C on Lipid Metabolism." *South African Journal of Nutrition (Supplement)* 61: 1651.

Lewin, S. 1976. *Vitamin C: Its Molecular Biology and Medical Potential.* Orlando, Fl. Academic Press.

Maas, J., G. Glesser, and L. Gottchalk. 1961. "Schizophrenia, Anxiety and Biochemical Factors." *Archives of General Psychiatry* 4: 109.

Man-Li S. Yew. 1973. "Recommended Daily Allowances for Vitamin C." *Proceedings of the National Academy of Sciences USA* 70: 969.

May C.D., C.T. Stewart, A. Hamilton, and R.J. Salmon. 1952. "Infection as a Cause of Folic Acid Deficiency and Megaloblastic Anemia." *American Journal of Diseases of Children* 84: 718.

McGanity, W.J., M. Fujino, and E. Dawson. 1967. "Nutritional Aspects of Gynecia Stress." *American Journal of Obstetrics and Gynecology* 97: 750.

Mowle, A. F. 1982. Ascorbate (Vit C) Utilization in Humans When Subjected to Moderate/Heavy Physiological Stress." *Australasian Nurses Journal* 11: 13.

_____. 1981. "To Run or Not to Run—That Is the Question and Reply. Ascorbate (Vit C) Utilization and Stressful Physical Exertion." *Australasian Nurses Journal* 10: 29.

Nandi, B.K., N. Subramanian, A.K. Majumder, and I.B. Chatterjee. 1974. "Effect of Ascorbic Acid on Detoxification of Histamine under Stress Conditions." *Biochemical Pharmacology* 23: 643.

Paré, W.P. 1968 "Effect of Duration of Environmental Stress on Stomach Ulceration and Adrenal Ascorbic Acid." *Psychological Reports* 23: 683.

_____. 1964. "The Effect of Chronic Environmental Stress on Stomach Ulceration, Adrenal Function and Consummatory Behavior in the Rat." *Journal of Psychology* 57: 143.

Pauling, L. 1976. "For the Best of Health—How Much Vitamin C?" *Pennsylvania Dental Journal* 49: 53.

_____. 1971. *Vitamin C and the Common Cold*. San Francisco: W.H. Freeman Co.

Pellitier, O. 1968. "Smoking and Vitamin C Levels in Humans." *American Journal of Clinical Nutrition* 21: (11) 1259.

Pfeiffer, C.C. 1975. *Mental and Elemental Nutrients*. New Canaan, Conn.: Keats.

Pohujani, S.M., S.M. Chittal, V.S. Raut, and U.K. Sheth. 1969. "Studies in Stress Induced Changes on Rats' Adrenals. Part III. Effect of Pre-treatment with Ascorbic Acid." *Indian Journal of Medical Research* 57: 1091.

Raineri, S. and J.H. Weisburger. 1975. "Reduction of Gastric Carcinogens with Ascorbic Acid." *Annals of the New York Academy of Sciences* 258: 181.

Schayer, R.W. 1962. "Role of Induced Histamine in Tourniquet Shock in Mice." *American Journal of Physiology* 203: 412.

Spittle, C.R. 1971. "Atherosclerosis and Vitamin C." *Lancet* 2: 1280.

Stone, I. 1976. "Smoker's Scurvy: Orthomolecular Preventive Medicine in Cigarette Smoking." *Journal of Orthomolecular Psychiatry* 5: 35.

Subramanian, N., B.K. Nandi, A.K. Majumder, and I.B. Chatterjee. 1973. "Role of l-Ascorbic Acid on Detoxification of Histamine." *Biochemical Pharmacology* 22: 167.

Whitehead, C.C., R. Blair, D.W. Bannister, A.J. Evans. 1975. "The Involvement of Dietary Fat and Vitamins, Stress, Litter and Starvation on the Incidence of the Fatty Liver and Kidney Syndrome in Chicks." *Research in Veterinary Science* 18: 100.

Willis, G.C. 1953. "Experimental Study of Intimal Ground Substance in Atherosclerosis." *Canadian Medical Association Journal* 69: 17.

Zaitsev, N.F., L.A. Myannikov, and M.B. Sheikman. 1964. Vliianie Askorbinovoi Kesloty na Raspridelenie Mechennogo 4-C -14-Kholesterina v Tkaniakl pri Eksperimental nom Ateroskleroze." *Kardiologiia* 4: 30.

Zkharova, Z.V. 1967. "Vliianie Stressa na Izmenenie Mineral'nogo i Amino-keslotnogo Obmena v Obyzvestlennykl Thaneakh Krep. Patologic Heskaia Fiziologiia I." *Eksperimentalnaia Terapiia (Moskva)* 11: 59.

CHAPTER 5

Adler, S., R.D. Lindeman, M.J. Yiengst, E. Beard, and N.W. Shock. 1968. "Effect of Acute Acid Loading on Urinary Acid Excretion by the Aging Human Kidney." *Journal of Laboratory and Clinical Medicine* 72: 278.

Altura, B.M. 1979. "Sudden-Death Ischemic Heart Disease and Dietary Magnesium Intake: Is the Target Site Coronary Vascular Smooth Muscle?" *Medical Hypotheses* 5: 843.

Altura, B.M., and B.T. Altura. 1981. "Role of Magnesium Ions in Contractility of Blood Vessels and Skeletal Muscles." *Magnesium Bulletin* la: 102.

_____. 1974. "Magnesium and Contraction of Arterial Smooth Muscle." *Microvascular Research* 7: 145.

Altura, B.M. and B.T. Altura 1978. "Magnesium and Vascular Tone and Reactivity." *Blood Vessels* 15:5.

Altura, B.T. 1980. "Type A Behavior and Coronary Vasospasm: A Possible Role of Hypomagnesemia." *Medical Hypotheses* 6: 753.

Beisel, W.R., and R.S. Pekarek. 1972. "Acute Stress and Trace Element Metabolism," In *International Review of Neurobiology*, edited by C.C. Pfeiffer, Suppl. 1, pp. 53–76. New York/London: Academic Press.

Chutkow, J.G. 1972. "Distribution of Magnesium and Calcium in Brains of Normal and Magnesium Deficient Rats." *Mayo Clinic Proceedings* 47: 647

Clamage, D.M., C.S. Sanford, and J. Vander. 1976. "Effects of Psychosocial Stimuli in Plasma Renin Activity in Rats." *American Journal of Physiology* 16: 127.

Classen, H.G. 1981. "Stress and Magnesium." *Artery* 9: 182.

Classen, H.G., P. Marquardt, M. Spath, and K.A. Schumacher. 1971. "Hypermagnesemia Following Exposure to Acute Stress." *Pharmacology* 5: 287.

Coburn, J.W., R.C. Reba, and F.N. Craig. 1966. "Effect of Potassium Depletion on Response to Acute Heat Exposure in Unacclimatized Man." *American Journal of Physiology* 211: 117.

Dyckner, T., and P.O. Wester. 1983. "Effect of Magnesium on Blood Pressure." *British Medical Journal* 286: 1847.

Flynn, A., W.J. Pories, W.H. Strain, and O.A. Hill. 1971. "Mineral Element Correlation with Adenohypophyseal-Adrenal Cortex Function and Stress." *Science* 173: 1035.

Grignolo, A., J.P. Koepke, and P.A. Obrist. 1982. "Renal Function, Heart Rate and Blood Pressure during Exercise and Avoidance in Dogs." *American Journal of Physiology* 242: R482.

Günther, T., H. Ising, and H. Merker. 1978. "Electrolyte- und Kollagengehalt im Rattenherzen bei chronischem Magnesium-Mangel und Stress." *Journal of Clinical Chemistry and Clinical Biochemistry* 16: 293.

Heroux, O., D. Peter, and A. Heggtveit. 1977. "Long-term Effect of Suboptimal Dietary Magnesium on Magnesium and Calcium Contents of Organs, on Cold Tolerance and on Life Span, and Its Pathological Consequences in Rats." *Journal of Nutrition* 107: 1640.

Himly, M.I., and G.G. Somjen. 1968. "Distribution and Tissue Uptake of Magnesium Related to Its Pharmacological Effects." *American Journal of Physiology* 214: 406.

Hofmann, P., P.O. Schwille, and R. Thun. 1979. "Hypocalcemia during Restraint Stress in Rats." *Research in Experimental Medicine (Berlin)* 175: 159.

Iampietro, P.F., M. Mager, and E.B. Green. 1961. "Some Physiological Changes Accompanying Tetany Induced by Exposure to Hot, Wet Conditions." *Journal of Applied Physiology* 16: 409.

Ising, H. 1981. "Interaction of Noise-induced Stress and Mg Decrease." *Artery* 9: 205.

John, T.M. and J.C. George. 1977. "Blood Levels of Cyclic AMP, Thyroxine, Uric Acid, Certain Metabolites and Electrolytes under Heat Stress and Dehydration in the Pigeon." *Archives Internationales de Physiologie et de Biochimie* 85: 571.

Leary, W.P., and A.J. Reyes. 1983. "Magnesium and Sudden Death." *South African Medical Journal* 64: 697.

Light, K.C., J.P. Koepke, P.A. Obrist, and P.W. Willis IV. 1983. "Psychological Stress Induces Sodium and Fluid Retention in Men at High Risk for Hypertension." *Science* 220: 429.

Louis, W.J. and S. Spector. 1975. "The Effect of Salt Intake and Adrenal Steroids on Blood Pressure in a Genetic Strain of Hypertensive Rats." *Clinical and Experimental Physiology and Pharmacology* Suppl. 2: 131.

Markoff, C.M., V.V. Bankova, and A.G. Kutcherenko. 1978. "Biosynthesis and Metabolism of Aldosterone during a Neurogenic Stress." *Problemy Endokrinologii (Moskva)* 24: 117.

Meneely, G.R., and H.D. Battarbee. 1976. "High Sodium–Low Potassium Environment and Hypertension." *American Journal of Cardiology* 38: 768.

Moore, F.D. 1953. "Bodily Changes in Surgical Convalescence: I. The Normal Sequence—Observations and Interpretations." *Annals of Surgery* 137: 289.

Newell, G.K., and R.E. Beauchene. 1975. "Effects of Dietary Calcium Level, Acid Stress and Age on Renal, Serum and Bone Responses of Rats." *Journal of Nutrition* 105: 1039.

Paré, W.P., and T.E. McCarthy. 1966. "Urinary Sodium and Potassium and Prolonged Environmental Stress." *The Journal of Genetic Psychology* 108: 135.

Prasad, A.S., ed. 1982. *Clinical Biochemical and Nutritional Aspects of Trace Elements*. New York: Alan R. Liss.

Raab, W., E. Bajusz, H. Kimura, and H.C. Herrlich. 1968. "Isolation, Stress, Myocardial Electrolytes, and Epinephrine Cardiotoxicity in Rats." *Proceedings of the Society of Experimental Biology and Medicine* 127: 142.

Rabie, E.F., and M. Radulovacki. 1971. "Variation in Calcium Content of Cerebrospinal Fluid after Excitation." *East African Medical Journal* 48: 100.

Reynaert, R., S., Marcus, M. DePaepe, and G. Peeters. 1976. "Influences of Stress, Age and Sex on Serum Growth Hormone and Free Fatty Acid Levels in Cattle." *Hormone and Metabolic Research* 8: 109.

Rosenberg, I.H., and N.W. Solomons, eds. 1984. *Absorption and Malabsorption of Mineral Nutrients*. New York: Alan R. Liss.

Sabbot, I., and A. Costin. 1974a. "Cold Stress Induced Changes in the Uptake and Distribution of Radiolabelled Magnesium in the Brain and Pituitary of the Rat." *Experientia* 30: 905.

_____. 1974b "Effect of Stress on the Uptake of Radiolabelled Calcium in the Pituitary Gland and the Brain of the Rat." *Journal of Neurochemistry* 22: 731.

Schwille, P.O., W. Schiller, M. Reitzenstein, and P. Hermanek. 1974. "Hyperglucagonemia, Hypocalcemia and Diminished Gastric Mucosal Blood Flow—Evidence for an Etiological Role in Stress Ulcer Formation of Rat." *Experientia* 30: 824.

Schwille, P.O., H. Steiner, N.M. Samberger, and W. Schillerer. 1965. "Role of Calcitoninn Stress Ulcer Formation of Various Rat Models. Preliminary Report." *Research in Experimental Medicine* 165: 291.

Seelig, M.S. 1974. "Magnesium Interrelationships in Ischemic Heart Disease: A Review." *American Journal of Clinical Nutrition* 27: 59.

Spigel, I.M., and A. Ramsay. 1969. "Excretory Electrolytes and Response to Stress in a Reptile." *Journal of Comparative and Physiological Psychology* 68: 18.

Steyn, A.G. 1975. "The Effects of Captivity Stress on the Blood Chemical Values of the Chacma Baboon (*Papio ursinus*)." *Laboratory Animals* 9: 111.

Thorn, G.W., D. Jenkins, and J.C. Laidlow. 1953. "The Adrenal Response to Stress in Man." *Recent Progress in Hormone Research* 8: 171.

Tigranian, R.A., L.L. Orloff, N.F. Kalita, N.A. Davydova, and E.A. Pavlova. 1980. "Changes of Blood Levels of Several Hormones, Catecholamines, Prostaglandins, Electrolytes and cAMP in Man during Emotional Stress." *Endocrinologia Experimentalis* 14: 101.

Tollersrud, S., B. Banstad and K. Flatlandsmo. 1971. "Effects of Physical Stress on Serum Enzymes and Other Blood Constituents in Sheep." *Acta Veterinaria Scandinavica* 12: 229.

Turlapaty, P.D.V.M., and B.M. Altura. 1980. "Magnesium Deficiency Produces Spasms of Coronary Arteries: Relationship to Etiology of Sudden Death Ischemic Heart Disease." *Science* 208: 198.

Wohler, W.H. 1972. "Shipping Stress in Cattle: Blood Chemistry." *Modern Veterinary Practicum* 53: 39.

Woodward, D.L., and D.J. Reed. 1969. "Effect of Magnesium Deficiency on Electrolyte Distribution in the Rabbit." *American Journal of Physiology* 217: 1477.

CHAPTER 6

Allaway, W.H., J. Kobota, F. Losee, and M. Roth. 1968. "Selenium, Molybdenum and Vanadium in Human Blood." *Archives of Environmental Health* 16: 342.

Armario, A., R. Flos, and J. Balasch. 1978. "Stress Simulation: ACTH and the Effect on Trace Metals in Liver and Spleen." *Revista Espanola de Fisiologia* 34: 395.

Balasch, J. and R. Flos. 1975. "Plasmatic Variations of Factors Related to Iron Metabolism in Stress." *Agressologie* 16: 89.

Ballantyne, G.H. 1983. "Rapid Drop in Serum Iron Concentration following Cholecystectomy. A Metabolic Response to Stress." *The American Surgeon* 49. 146.

Bonfils, S., G. Rossi, and A. Lambling. 1958. "Stress for the Production of Ulcers." *Revue Francaise D'Etudes Cliniques et Biologiques (Paris)* 3: 977.

Brady, F.O. 1981. "Synthesis of Rat Hepatic Zinc Thioneine in Response to the Stress of Sham Operation." *Life Sciences* 28: 1647.

Brunia, C.H.M., and G. Buyze. 1972. "Serum Copper Levels and Epilepsy." *Epilepsia* 13: 621.

Calautti, P., G. Moschini, B.M. Stievano, L. Tomio, F. Calzavora, and G. Perona. 1980. "Serum Selenium Levels in Malignant Lymphoproliferative Diseases." *Scandinavian Journal of Haematology* 24: 63.

Canfield, W.K., and R.J. Dorsy. 1976. "Chrominum and Diabetes in the Aged." *The Biomedical Role of Trace Elements in Aging.* Davis, and Neithamer, edited by Hsu. St Petersburg, Fla. Eckerd College.

Carlson, H.E. 1984. "Inhibition of Prolactin and Growth Hormone Secretion by Nickel." *Life Sciences* 35: 1747.

Chandra, R.K. 1984. "Excessive Intake of Zinc Impairs Immune Responses." *Journal of the American Medical Association* 252: 1443.

———. 1980. "Single Nutrient Deficiency and Cell-mediated Immune Responses." *American Journal of Clinical Nutrition* 33: 736.

———. 1975. "Impaired Immunocompetence Associated with Iron Deficiency." *Journal of Pediatrics* 86: 899.

Chandra, R.K., B. Au, G. Woodford, and P. Hyam. 1977. "Iron Status, Immuno-competence and Susceptibility to Infection." In *Ciba Foundation Symposium on Iron Metabolism* p. 249. Amsterdam: Elsevier.

Chandra, S.V., P.K. Seth, and J.K. Mankeshwar. 1974. "Manganese Poisoning: Clinical and Biochemical Observations." *Environmental Research* 7: 374.

Chandra, S.V., G.S. Shukla, and R.C. Murthy. 1979. "Effect of Stress on the Response of Rat Brain to Manganese." *Toxicology and Applied Pharmacology* 47: 603.

Chesters, J.K. 1978. "Biochemical Functions of Zinc in Animals." *World Review of Nutrition and Dietetics* 32: 135.

Chesters, J.K., and M. Will. 1981. "Measurement of Zinc Flux through Plasma in Normal and Endotoxin-stressed Pigs and the Effects of Zn Supplementation during Stress." *British Journal of Nutrition* 46: 119.

Cho, C.H., and C.W. Ogle. 1978. "Correlative Study of the Antiulcer Effects of Zinc Sulfate in Stressed Rats." *European Journal of Pharmacology* 48: 97.

———. 1977. "The Effects of Zinc Sulfate on Vagal-induced Mast Cell Changes and Ulcers in the Rat Stomach." *European Journal of Pharmacology* 43: 315.

Cho, C.H., C.J. Pfeiffer, and A. Cheema. 1980. "Studies of Zinc and Histamine on Lysosomal Fragility: Possible Role in Stress Ulceration." *Pharmacology Biochemistry and Behavior* 13: 41.

Corrigal W., A.C. Dalgarno, and R.B. Williams. 1976. "Modulation of Plasma, Copper and Zinc Concentrations by Disease States in Ruminants." *Veterinary Record* 99: 396.

Cox, R.P., and A. Ruckenstern. 1971. "Studies on the Mechanism of Hormonal Stimulation of Zinc Uptake in Human Cell Cultures." *Journal of Cellular Physiology* 77: 71.

Curzon, G., and A.R. Green. 1969. "Effects of Immobilization on Rat Liver Tryptophan Pyrrolase and Brain 5-HT Metabolism." *British Journal of Pharmacology* 37: 689.

Curzon, G., M.H. Joseph, and P.J. Knott. 1972. "Effect of Immobilization and Food Deprivation on Rat Brain Tryptophan Metabolism." *Journal of Neurochemistry* 19: 1967.

Dormer, R.L., A.L. Kerbey, M. McPherson, S. Manley, S.J.H. Ashcroft, J.G. Schofield, and P.J. Randle. 1973. "The Effect of Nickel on Secretory Systems. Studies on the Release of Amylase, Insulin and Growth Hormones." *Journal of Biochemistry* 140: 135.

Falchuk, K.H. 1977. "Effect of Acute Disease and ACTH on Serum Zinc Proteins." *New England Journal of Medicine* 296: 1129.

Feldthusen, U., V. Larsen, and N.A. Lassen. 1953. "Serum Iron and Operative Stress." *Acta Medica Scandinavica* 147: 311.

Fernandes, G., M. Nair, K. Onoe, T. Tanaka, R. Floyd, and R.A. Good. 1979. "Impairment of Cell-mediated Immunity Functions by Dietary Zinc Deficiency in Mice." *Proceedings of the National Academy of Sciences USA* 76: 457.

Fitzsimons, E.J., and K. Kaplan. 1980. "Rapid Drop in Serum Iron Concentrations in Myocardial Infarction." *American Journal of Clinical Pathology* 73: 552.

Fitzsimons, E.J., and S.R. Levine. 1983. "Rapid Drop in Serum Iron Concentration Associated with Stress." *The American Journal of the Medical Sciences* 283: 12.

Flos, R., and A. Armario. 1978. "Stress Stimulation and Iron Metabolism: Adrenaline Administration." *Revista Espanola de Fisiologia* 34: 167.

Flynn, A., W.J. Pories, W.H. Strain, and O.A. Hill. Jr. 1971a. "Mineral Element Correlation with Adenohypophyseal–Adrenal Cortex Function and Stress." *Science* 173: 1035.

Flynn, A., W.J. Pories, W.H. Strain, O.A. Hill, Jr., and R.B. Fratianne. 1971b. "Rapid Serum-Zinc Depletion Associated with Corticosteroid Therapy." *Lancet* 2: 1169.

Flynn, A., W.H. Strain, and W.J. Pories. 1972. "Corticotropin Dependency on Zinc Ions." *Biochemical and Biophysical Research Communications* 46: 1113.

Fracker, P.J., P. Depasquale-Jardieu, C.M. Zwicki, and R.W. Leucke. 1978. "Regeneration of T-cell Helper Function in Zinc-Deficient Adult Mice." *Proceedings of the National Academy of Sciences USA* 75: 5660.

Gross, R.L., N. Osdin, L. Fong, and P.M. Newberne. 1979. "Depressed Immunological Function in zinc-deprived Rats as Measured by Mitogen Response of Spleen, Thymus and Peripheral Blood." *American Journal of Clinical Nutrition* 32: 1260.

Hallbook, T., and H. Hedelin. 1977. "Zinc Metabolism and Surgical Trauma." *British Journal of Surgery* 64: 271.

Hambidge, K.M., and W. Droegemueller. 1974. "Changes in Plasma and Hair Concentrations of Zinc, Copper, Chromium and Manganese during Pregnancy." *Obstetrics and Gynecology Annual* 44: 666.

Helzlsouer, K.J. 1983. "Selenium and Cancer Prevention." *Seminars in Oncology* 10: 305.

Henkin, R.I., and F.R. Smith. 1972. "Zinc and Copper Metabolism in Acute Viral Hepatitis." *American Journal of the Medical Sciences* 264: 401.

Herring, B.W., B.S. Leavell, L.M. Paixav, and J.H. Yoe. 1960. "Trace Metals in Human Plasma and Red Blood Cells. Observations of Normal Subject." *American Journal of Clinical Nutrition* 8: 846.

Hsu, J.M. 1979. "Current Knowledge on Zinc, Copper and Chromium in Aging." *World Review of Nutrition and Dietetics* 33: 42.

Kincaid, R.L., W.J. Miller, R.P. Gentry, M.W. Neathery, D.L. Hampton, and J.W. Lassiter. 1976. "The Effect of Endotoxin upon Zinc Retention and Intracellular Liver Distribution in Rats." *Nutrition Reports International* 13: 65.

Klevay, L.M. 1983. "Copper and Ischemic Heart Disease." *Biological Trace Element Research* 5: 245.

Kluger, M.J., and B.A. Rothenburg. 1979. "Fever and Reduced Iron. Their Interactions as a Host Defense Response to Bacterial Infection." *Science* 203: 374.

Labella, F.S., R. Dular, P. Lemon, S. Vivian, and G. Queen. 1973a. "Prolactin Secretion Is Specifically Inhibited by Nickel." *Nature* 245: 330.

_____. 1973b "Pituitary Hormone Releasing or Inhibiting Activity of Metal Ions Present on Hypothalamic Extracts." *Biochemical and Biophysical Research Communications* 52: 786.

Lahey, M.E., C.J. Gubler, G.E. Cartwright, and M.M. Wintrobe. 1953. "Studies on Copper Metabolism. VI. Blood Copper in Normal Human Subjects." *Journal of Clinical Investigation* 32: 322.

Lindeman, R.D., R.G. Bottomley, R.L. Cornelison, and L.A. Jacobs. 1972. "Influence of Acute Tissue Injury on Zinc Metabolism in Man." *Journal of Laboratory and Clinical Medicine* 79: 452.

MacDougall, L.G., R. Anderson, G.M. McNab, and J. Katz. 1975. "Immune Response in Iron-deficient Children. Impaired Cellular Defense Mechanisms with Altered Hormonal Components." *Journal of Pediatrics* 86: 833.

McConnell, K.P., R.M. Jayer, K.I. Bland, and A.J. Blotcky. 1980. "The Relationship of Dietary Selenium and Breast Cancer." *Journal of Surgical Oncology* 15: 67.

Mertz, W., E.E. Roginski, and K. Schwartz. 1961. "Effect of Trivalent Chromium Complex on Glucose Uptake by Epididymal Fat Tissue of Rats." *Journal of Biological Chemistry* 236: 318.

Mertz, W., and E.E. Roginski. 1969. "Effects of Chromium III Supplementation on Growth and Survival under Stress in Rats Fed Low Protein Diets." *Journal of Nutrition* 97: 531.

Pekarek, R.S., G.S. Burghen, P.J. Bartelloni, F.M. Calia, K.A. Bostian, and W.R. Beisel. 1970. "The Effect of Live Attenuated Venezuelan Equine Encephalomyelitis Virus Vaccine on Serum Iron, Zinc and Copper Concentrations in Man." *Journal of Laboratory and Clinical Medicine* 76: 293.

Prasad, A.S., I.E. Dreosti, and B.S. Hetzel. 1982. eds. *Clinical Applications of Recent Advances in Zinc Metabolism*. New York: Alan R. Liss.

Reeves, P.G., S.G. Frissell, and B.L. O'Dell. 1977. "Response of Serum Corticosterone to ACTH and Stress in the Zinc-deficient Rat." *Proceedings of the Society for Experimental Biology and Medicine* 156: 500.

Sandstead, H.H., A.S. Prasad, A.R. Schulert, Z. Farid, A. Miale, Jr. S. Bassily, and W.J. Darby. *In* A Prasad (Ed.) "Zinc Metabolism" pp. 304, Thomas Springfield, Il.

Schloen, L.H., G. Fernandes, J.A. Garofalo, and R.A. Good. 1979. "Nutrition

Immunity and Cancer—A review—Part II. Zinc, Immune Function and Cancer." *Clinical Bulletin* 9: 63.

Schwartz, K. 1977. "Essentiality versus Toxicity of Metals." In *Clinical Chemistry and Chemical Toxicology of Metals*, edited by S.S. Brown. Amsterdam: Elsevier.

Spallholz, J.E., J.L. Martin, M.L. Gerlach, and R.H. Heinzerling. 1975. "Injectable Selenium: Effect in the Primary Immune Response of Mice." *Proceedings of the Society of Experimental Biology and Medicine* 148: 37.

Sugawara, N., C. Sugawara, N. Maehara, T. Sadamato, I. Harabuchi, and K. Yamamura. 1983. "Effect of Acute Stresses on Zn-Thionein Production in Rat Liver." *European Journal of Applied Physiology* 51: 365.

Sunderman, F.W., Jr., S. Nomoto, A.M. Pradhan, H. Levine, S.H. Bernstein, and R. Hirsch. 1970. "Increased Concentrations of Serum Nickel after Acute Myocardial Infarction." *New England Journal of Medicine* 283: 896.

Syrkis, I., and I. Machtey. 1973. "Hypoferremia in Acute Myocardial Infarction." *Journal of the American Geriatric Society* 21: 28.

Vikbladh, I. 1951. "Studies on Zinc in Blood." *Scandinavian Journal of Clinical and Laboratory Investigation*. Suppl. 2: 3.

Wegner, T.N., D.E. Ray, C.D. Lox, and G.H. Stott. 1972. "Effect of Stress on Serum Zinc and Plasma Corticoids in Dairy Cattle." *Journal of Dairy Science* 56: 748.

Weinberg, E.D. 1978. "Iron and Infection." *Microbiology Reviews* 42: 45.

_____. 1975. "Nutritional Immunity. Hosts Attempt to Withold Iron from Microbial Invaders." *Journal of the American Medical Association* 231: 39.

_____. 1974. "Iron and Susceptibility to Infectious Diseases." *Science* 184: 952.

Weisenberg, R.C., G.G. Boisy, and E.W. Taylor. 1968. "The colchicine-binding Protein of Mammalian Brain and Its Relation to Microtubules." *Biochemistry* 7: 4466.

Willett, W., B.F. Polk, C. Hames, J.S. Morris, M.J. Stampfer, S. Pressel, B. Rosner, J.O. Taylor, and K. Schneider. 1983. "Prediagnostic Serum Selenium and the Risk of Cancer." *Lancet* 2: 130.

CHAPTER 7

Asterita, M.F. 1985. *The Physiology of Stress: With Special Reference to the Neuroendocrine System.* New York: Human Sciences Press.

Beattie, A.D., M.R. Moore, A. Goldberg, M.J.W. Finlayson, J.I. Graham, E.M. Mackie, J.C. Naire, T.A. McLaren, R.M. Murdock, and G.T. Steuart. 1975. "Role of Chronic Low Level Lead Exposure in the Aetiology of Mental Retardation." *Lancet* 1: 589.

Berg, L.R., Jon O. Nordstrom, and L.E. Ousterhout. 1980. "Prevention of Chick Growth Depression due to Dietary Lead by Increased Dietary Calcium and Phosphorus Levels." *Poultry Science* 59: 1860.

Crapper, D.R., S.S. Krishman, and A.J. Dalton. 1973. "Brain Aluminum Distribution and Experimental Distribution and Experimental Neurofibrillary Degeneration." *Science* 180: 511.

Eck, P. 1981. *The Healthview Newsletter.* Issues 27–29. Charlottesville, Va.

Kopeloff, L., S. Barrera, N. Kopeloff. 1942. "Recurrent Convulsive Seizures in Animals Produced by Immunologic and Chemical Means." *American Journal of Psychiatry* 98: 881.

Laporte, R.E., and E.E. Talbott. 1978. "Effects of Low Levels of Lead Exposure on Cognitive Function—A Review." *Archives of Environmental Health* 33: 236.

Malter, R.F. "Implications of a Bio-Nutritional Approach to the Diagnosis, Treatment, and Cost of L.D." *Somatics* Autumn-Winter 1984–85. p. 38.

Morgan, J.M. 1970. "Cadmium and Zinc Abnormalities in Bronchogenic Carcinoma." *Cancer* 25: 1394.

National Research Council. 1971. *Airborne Lead in Perspective*. Washington D.C.: National Academy of Sciences, National Academy of Engineering.

_____. 1980. *Mineral Tolerances of Domestic Animals*. Washington, D.C.: National Academy of Sciences.

Passwater, R.A. and E.M. Cranton. 1983. *Trace Elements, Hair Analysis and Nutrition*. New Canaan, Conn.: Keats Publishing Co.

Richie, D. 1984. "Stress Induced by Toxic Elements." In *Stress Management Manual*. Mundelein Ill. International Minerals and Chemical Corporation, Animal Health and Nutrition Division.

Sell, J.L. 1974. "Metabolism and Toxicity of Cadmium and Mercury." Minnesota Nutrition Conference, *Proceedings* 1.

Selye, H. 1976. *Stress in Health and Disease*. Reading, Mass: Butterworths.

Watson, G. 1972. *Nutrition and Your Mind*. New York: Bantam Books.

Zarkowsky, H. 1975. "Chronic Low-Level Lead Exposure and Mental Retardation." *Lancet* 2: 1087.

CHAPTER 8

Arola, L.L., A. Palou, X. Remesar, E. Herrera, and M. Alemany. 1980. "Effect of Stress and Sampling Site on Metabolic Concentration in Rat Plasma." *Archives Internationales de Physiologie et de Biochimie* 88: 99.

Benes, V., and V. Hrubes. 1968. "Serum Free Fatty Acid Level after an Experimentally Induced Emotional Stress and Its Modification by Nicotonic Acid in Rats with Different Characteristics of Higher Nervous Activity." *Activitas Nervosa Superior (Praha)* 10: 395.

Berger, D.F., J.J. Starzec, E.B. Mason, and W. DeVito. 1980. "The Effects of Differential Psychological Stress on Plasma Cholesterol Levels in Rats." *Psychosomatic Medicine* 42: 481.

Bogdonoff, M.D., E.H. Estes, and D. Trout. 1959. "Acute Effect of Psychogenic Stimuli upon Plasma Nonesterfied Fatty Acid." *Proceedings of the Society of Experimental Biology and Medicine* 100: 503.

Brooks, G.W., and E. Mueller. 1966. "Serum Urate Concentrations among University Professors." *Journal of the American Medical Association* 195: 431.

Carlson, L.A., L. Levi, L. Orö. 1968. "Plasma Lipids and Urinary Excretion of Catecholamines in Man during Experimentally Induced Emotional Stress and Their Modification by Nicotinic Acid." *Journal of Clinical Investigation* 47: 1795.

Cathey, C.W., R.F. Redmond, and S. Wolf. 1957. "Serum Cholesterol, Diet and Stress in Patients with Coronary Artery Disease." (Abstract.) *Journal of Clinical Investigation* 36: 897.

Chait, A., J.D. Brunzell, D.G. Johnson, J.W. Benson, P. Warner, J.P. Palmer, J.J. Albers, J.W. Ensinck, and E.L. Biermann. 1979. "Reduction of Plasma Triglyceride Concentration by Acute Stress in Man." *Metabolism* 28: 553.

Dayton S. 1976. "Polyunsaturated Fats." In *Nutrition and Cardiovascular Disease* edited by E.B. Feldman. New York: Appleton-Century Crofts.

Dimsdale, J.E., and A. Herd. 1982. "Variability of Plasma Lipids in Response to Emotional Arousal." *Psychosomatic Medicine* 44: 413.

Dolkas, C.B., H.A. Leon, and M. Chackerian. 1971. "Short Term Response of Insulin, Glucose, Growth Hormone and Corticosterone to Acute Vibration in Rats." *Aerospace Medicine* 42: 723.

Dreyfuss, F., and J.W. Czaczkes. 1959. "Blood Cholesterol and Uric Acid of Healthy Medical Students under Stress of an Examination." *Archives of Internal Medicine* 103: 708.

Dunn, J.P. 1963. "Social Class Gradient of Serum Uric Acid Levels in Males." *Journal of the American Medical Association* 185: 431.

Euler, U.S. 1964. "Quantitation of Stress by Catecholamine Analysis." *Clinical Pharmacology and Therapeutics* 5: 398.

Feigelson, E.B., W.W. Pfaff, A. Karmen, and D. Steinberg. 1961. "The Role of Plasma Free Fatty Acids in Development of Fatty Liver." *Journal of Clinical Investigation* 40: 2171.

Feldman, E.B. 1976. "Saturated Fats." In *Nutrition and Cardiovascular Disease* edited by E.B. Feldman. New York: Appleton Century-Crofts.

Francis, K.T. 1979. "Psychologic Correlates of Serum Indicators of Stress in Man: A Longitudinal Study." *Psychosomatic Medicine* 41: 617.

Friedman, M., and S.O. Byers. 1960. "Effects of Epinephrine and Norepinephrine on Lipid Metabolism of the Rat." *American Journal of Physiology* 199: 995.

Friedman, M., R.H. Rosemman, and V. Carroll. 1958. "Changes in the Serum Cholesterol and Blood Clotting Time in Man Subjected to Cyclic Variation of Occupational Stress." *Circulation* 17: 852.

Gittleman, B., L. Shatin, M.L. Bierenbaum, A.I. Flesichman, and T. Hayton. 1968. "Effects of Quantified Stressful Stimuli on Blood Lipids in Man. *Journal of Nervous and Mental Disease* 147: 196.

Gordon, P.V., and R.S. Gordon. 1959. "Rapid Increase in Plasma Unesterified Fatty Acids in Man during Fear." *Journal of Psychosomatic Research* 4: 5.

Grundy, S.M., and A.C. Griffin. 1959a. "Effects of Periodic Mental Stress on Serum and Cholesterol Levels." *Circulation* 19: 496.

———. 1959b. "Relationship of Periodic Mental Stress on Serum Lipoprotein and Cholesterol Levels." *Journal of the American Medical Association* 171: 1794.

Hall, J.B., and D.A. Brown. 1979. "Plasma Glucose and Lactic Acid Alterations in Response to a Stressful Exam." *Biological Psychology* 8: 179.

Havel, R.J., and A. Goldfien. 1959. "The Role of the Sympathetic Nervous System in the Metabolism of Free Fatty Acids." *Journal of Lipid Research* 1: 102.

Henry, J.P., N.L. Ely, P.M. Stephens, H.L. Ratcliffe, C.A. Santisteban, and A.P. Shapiro. 1971. "The Role of Psychosocial Factors in the Development of Arteriosclerosis in CBA Mice. Observations on the Heart, Kidney and Aorta." *Arteriosclerosis* 14: 203.

Hoffel, G., and M. Moriarty. 1924. "The Effect of Fasting on the Metabolism of Epileptic Children." *American Journal of Diseases of Children* 28: 16.

John, T.M. and J.C. George. 1977. "Blood Levels of Cyclic AMP, Thyroxine, Uric Acid, Certain Metabolites and Electrolytes under Heat Stress and Dehydration in the Pigeon." *Archives Internationales de Physiologie et de Biochimie* 85: 571.

Kahn, A.U., R.B. Forneey, and F.W. Hughes. 1964. "Stress of Shocking Stimulus on Plasma Free Fatty Acids in Rats." *Archives Internationales de Pharmacodynamie et de Therapie* 3: 459.

Kameyama, T., T. Nebeshima, and H. Nagata. 1981. "Hypoglycemia in Mice Exposed to an Environment of High Temperature and Humidity." *Research Communications in Chemical Pathology and Pharmacology* 32: 261.

Keys A. 1970. ed. "Coronary Heart Disease in Seven Countries." AHA Monograph No. 29. *Circulation* 41. (Suppl. 1).

Levi, L. 1963. "The Urinary Output of Adrenalin and Noradrenalin during Experimentally Induced Emotional Stress in Clinically Different Groups. A Preliminary Report." *Acta Psychotherapeutica* 11: 8.

Mann, G.V., and H.S. White. 1953. "The Influence of Stress on Plasma Cholesterol Levels." *Metabolism* 2: 47.

Mayes, P.A. 1962. "Blood Glucose and Plasma Unesterified Fatty Acids Changes Induced by the Stress of an Emergency Situation." *Experientia* 18: 541.

Mueller, P.S., J.M. Davis, W.E. Bunney, Jr., H. Weil-Malherbe, and P.V. Cardon. 1970. "Plasma Free Fatty Acids Concentration in Depressive Illness." *Archives of General Psychiatry* 22: 216.

Painter, N.S., A.Z. Almeida, and K.W. Colebourne. 1972. "Unprocessed Bran in Treatment of Diverticular Disease of the Colon." *British Medical Journal* 2: 137.

Paré, W.P., B. Rothfeld, K.E. Isom, and A. Varady. 1973. "Cholesterol Synthesis and Metabolism as a Function of Unpredictable Shock Stimulation." *Physiology and Behavior* 11: 107.

Pfeiffer, C.C., V. Iliev, R.E. Nichols, and A.A. Sugerman. 1969. "The Serum Urate Level Reflects Degree of Stress." *The Journal of Clinical Pharmacology* 9: 384.

Rahe, R.H., and R.J. Arthur. 1967. "Stressful Underwater Demolition Training." *Journal of the American Medical Association* 202: 1052.

Rahe, R.H., R.T. Rubin, R.J. Arthur, and B.R. Clark. 1968. "Serum Uric Acid and Cholesterol Variability." *Journal of the American Medical Association* 206: 2875.

Rahe, R.H., R.T. Rubin, E.K. Gunderson, and R.J. Arthur. 1971. "Psychologic Correlates of Serum Cholesterol in Man, a Longitudinal Study." *Psychosomatic Medicine* 33: 399.

Reilly, P.E.B., and L.G. Chandrasena. 1979. "Indices of Stress in Housed Experimental Sheep." *Research in Veterinary Science* 27: 250.

Reynaert, R., S. Marcus, M. De Paepe, and G. Peeters. 1976. "Influences of Stress, Age and Sex on Serum Growth Hormone and Free Fatty Acid Levels in Cattle." *Hormone and Metabolic Research* 8: 109.

Rothfeld, B., A. Karmen and C. Hunter. 1970. "Some Effect of CPIB in the Rat." *Biochemical Medicine* 3: 344.

Rothfeld, B., W.P. Paré, A. Varady, Jr., K.E. Isom, and A. Karmen. 1973. "The Effects of Environmental Stress on Cholesterol Synthesis and Metabolism." *Biochemical Medicine* 7: 292.

Sloane, R.B., A. Habib, M.B. Eveson, and R.W. Payne. 1961. "Some Behavorial and Other Correlates of Cholesterol Metabolism." *Journal of Psychosomatic Research* 5: 183.

Stetten, D. 1959. "Gout." *Perspectives in Biology and Medicine* 2: 185.

Stetten, D., and J.Z. Hearon. 1959. "Intellectual Level Measured by Army Classification Battery and Serum Uric Acid Concentration." *Science* 129: 1737.

Steyn, A.G. 1975. "The Effects of Captivity Stress on the Blood Chemical Values of the Chacma Baboon (*Papio ursinus*)." *Laboratory Animals* 9: 111.

Taggart, P., and M. Carruthers. 1971. "Endogenous Hyperlipidaemia Induced by Emotional Stress of Racing Driving." *Lancet* 1: 363.

Taggart, P., M. Carruthers, and W. Somerville. 1973. "Electrocardiogram, Plasma Catecholamines and Lipids and Their Modification by Oxprenolol when Speaking Before an Audience." *Lancet* 2: 341.

Thomas, C.B., and E.A. Murphy. 1958. "Further Studies on Cholesterol Levels in the Johns Hopkins Medical Students, the Effect of Stress at Examination." *Journal of Chronic Diseases* 8: 661.

Tigranian, R.A., L.L. Orloff, N.F. Kalita, N.A. Davydova, and E.A. Pavlova. 1980. "Changes of Blood Levels of Several Hormones, Catecholamines, Prostaglandins, Electrolytes and cAMP in Man during Emotional Stress." *Endocrinologia Experimentalis* 14: 101.

Tollersrud, S. 1970. "Heat Stability of Serum Lactate Dehydrogenase and Its Isoenzymes in Young and Adult Cattle and Sheep. Evaluation of a Relative Heat Stability Test and Serum Determination of *alpha*-Hydroxybutyrate Dehydrogenase in Diagnostic Work." *Acta Veterinaria Scandinavica* 11: 510.

_____. 1969. "Stability of Some Serum enzymes in Sheep, Cattle and Swine during Storage at Different Temperatures." *Acta Veterinaria Scandinavica* 10: 359.

Tollersrud, S., B. Banstad, and K. Flatlandsmo. 1971. "Effects of Physical Stress on Serum Enzymes and Other Blood Constituents in Sheep." *Acta Veterinaria Scandinavica* 12: 220.

Válek, J., and E. Kuln. 1970. "Stress-induced Changes of Carbohydrates and Lipid Metabolism in Coronary Disease (CHD)." *Psychotherapy and Psychosomatics* 18: 275. (Recent Research in Psychosomatics. 8th European Conference on Psychosomatic Research, Knokke, 1970.)

Wertlake, P.T., A.A. Wilcox, M.I. Haley, and J.E. Peterson. 1958. "Relationship of Mental and Emotional Stress to Serum cholesterol Levels." *Proceedings of the Society of Experimental Biology and Medicine* 97: 163.

Wohler, W.H. Jr., 1972. "Shipping Stress in Cattle: Blood Chemistry." *Modern Veterinary Practicum* 53: 39.

CHAPTER 9

Balmer, J., and D.B. Zilversmit. 1974. "Effects of Dietary Roughage on Cholesterol Absorption, Cholesterol Turnover and Steroid Excretion in the Rat." *Journal of Nutrition* 104: 319.

Kim, B.I. 1963. "Studies on Effects of Ginseng and Other Drugs upon the Tolerance of Mice to Cold." *Korean Medical Journal* 8: 107.

Kim, C.C. 1966. "Studies on the Effects of Temperatures and Some Drugs on the Tolerance and the Serum Protein of Mice Exposed to Positive Radial Acceleration." *Korean Medical Journal* 11: 51.

Kim, C., C.C. Kim, M.S. Kim, C.Y. Hu, and J.S. Rhe. 1970. "Influence of Ginseng on the Stress Mechanism." *Lloydia* 33:43.

Trowell, H. 1976. "Definition of Dietary Fiber and Hypothesis That It Is a Protective Factor in Certain Diseases." *American Journal of Clinical Nutrition* 29: 417.

Trowell, H. 1972. "Ischemic Heart Disease and Dietary Fiber." *American Journal of Clinical Nutrition* 25: 926.

Wood, W.B., B.L. Roh, and R.P. White. 1964. "Cardiovascular Actions of Panax Ginseng in Dogs."*Japanese Journal of Pharmacology* 14: 284.

Yoon, S.R. 1960. "5-Hydroxytryptamine and Panax Ginseng on the Mobility of the Stomach and Intestine." *Korean Medical Journal* 5: 832.

GLOSSARY

Acetylcholine Important neurotransmitter of the autonomic nervous system and also the brain.

Acidophilus Supplementary food claimed to be a good source of intestinal bacteria.

ACTH See adrenocorticotropin hormone.

Adenosine triphosphate Compound of adenosine with three phosphoric acids at the 5' position.

ADH See antidiuretic hormone.

Adipose tissue Tissue that is composed of and stores fat.

Adrenal Cortex Portion of the adrenal gland that secretes many substances, including sex hormones, the glucocorticoids, which influence protein and carbohydrate metabolism, and the mineralocorticoids, which influence electrolyte metabolism.

Adrenal gland Triangular gland situated adjacent to and covering the superior portion of each kidney.

Adrenal medulla Portion of the adrenal gland that secretes the hormones epinephrine and norepinephrine.

Adrenaline Another name for epinephrine.

Adrenocorticotropin Hormone secreted by the pituitary gland whose main function is to control glucocorticoid secretion by the adrenal gland. It is secreted during acute and chronic stress.

-aemia See -emia.

Alanine Nonessential amino acid.

Aldosterone Hormone secreted by the adrenal cortex that plays a role in the regulation of water and electrolyte (sodium and potassium) balance in the body.

Alfalfa Leguminous plant that is considered to be a good source of several vitamins and minerals.

***alpha*-Tocopherol** The most biologically active and potent form of vitamin E.

Aluminum   Silver-white metallic element. It is widely used in several commercial products as well as in industry.

Amenorrhea   Abnormal or suppressed menstruation. It normally occurs before puberty, after menopause, and during pregnancy and lactation.

Amino Acids   Organic substances of small molecular size that contain an amino group ($-NH_2$) at one end and a carboxyl group ($-COOH$) at the other end. Amino acids are the structural units of proteins.

Anabolism   The building up of body tissue.

Anemia   A condition in which there is a decrease in the hemoglobin content or a decrease in the number of circulating red blood cells or both. There are several types of anemias, each classified according to morphology, hemoglobin concentration, and etiology.

Angina   A disease characterized by spasmodic attacks of intense pain.

Anion   An ion with a negative charge.

Anorexia   Loss of appetite.

Antibody   Protein substance produced by the body usually in response to the presence of an antigen that has entered the circulation.

Anticoagulant   Substance that prevents or delays the clotting of blood.

Antidiuretic hormone   Hormone secreted by the posterior pituitary gland. It plays a role in water reabsorption by the distal tubules of the kidney.

Antimony   Metallic element. Many of its compounds are used in alloys and in various medicines.

Antioxidant   Substance that prevents oxidation and thus inhibits the degeneration of other materials and tissues through oxidative processes.

Antirachitic   Substance used in the treatment and prevention of rickets.

Antiulcer vitamin   Substance thought to prevent ulcer formation. It has also been called vitamin U or cabagin.

Arachidonic acid   Polyunsaturated fatty acid that is a biosynthetic precursor of several biological compounds necessary for body function.

Arginine   Nonessential amino acid obtained from the degradation of protein products.

Arrhythmia   Irregular heartbeat caused by any number of physiological or pathological disturbances.

Arsenic Metallic element considered to be highly toxic. It is used commercially in the manufacture of several dyes and medicines.

Arterial blood pressure The pressure the blood exerts on the walls of the arteries.

Arteriosclerosis Name given to several conditions characterized by a hardening or loss of elasticity of blood vessel walls, especially the arteries.

Arthritis Inflammation of the joints usually accompanied by pain.

Articular rheumatism Refers to various conditions of pain sometimes accompanied by other symptoms which are of articular origin.

Ascorbic acid Another name for vitamin C.

Asparagine Nonessential amino acid.

Aspartic acid Nonessential amino acid.

Asthma Disorder characterized by either bronchial spasms or swelling of the mucous membranes in the respiratory tract.

Ataxia Inability to coordinate muscular movement.

Atherosclerosis Form of arteriosclerosis characterized by local accumulations of lipid materials in blood vessel walls.

ATP See adenosine triphosphate.

Autism Mental state or condition in which reality is focused within, on one's ego.

Autonomic nervous system The part of the nervous system that controls involuntary functions, glandular secretory activity, and smooth muscle function. It includes the sympathetic and parasympathetic nervous systems.

Barium Soft metallic element that is a member of the alkaline earth group.

Baroreceptors Receptors located in different areas of the body that respond to changes in stretch of a tissue, hence they are sensitive to pressure changes.

Bee propolis Resinous substance produced by bees that serves as an antibiotic for them. There are some claims that it may have a similar effect in humans.

Beriberi Deficiency disease that can result from a lack of proper nutrition. It occurs specifically because of a lack of vitamin B_1 (thiamine) in the diet.

Beryllium Metallic element heavily used in industry.

***Beta*-Hydroxyglutamic acid** Nonessential amino acid.

Biotin This substance was formally known as vitamin H. It is now considered to be a member of the B complex vitamin family.

Bismuth Metallic element. Many of its salts are used as antiseptics and astringents.

Blackstrap molasses Supplementary food that is claimed to be a rich source of many nutrients, including several vitamins and minerals.

Blood pressure The pressure the blood exerts on the walls of the blood vessels.

Bone meal Supplementary food that consists of finely ground bone. It is considered to be a good source of both calcium and phosphorus.

Boron Nonmetallic element found commonly in nature in a compound called boric acid.

Brewers yeast Supplementary food that is a good source of many nutrients, including several vitamins and minerals.

Bromine Nonmetallic element that is liquid at room temperature. It belongs to the group of nonmetals called the halogens.

Cabagin See antiulcer vitamin.

Cadmium Metallic element. Its compounds are widely used in industry.

Calcitonin Hormone secreted by the thyroid gland that aids in regulating the levels of calcium in the blood. Also known as thyrocalcitonin.

Calcium Metallic element with several important physiological functions.

Calcium pantothenate Another name for vitamin B_5.

Carbohydrates Class of organic compounds that have the same ratio of hydrogen and oxygen atoms as that found in water and can be represented by the formula $C_x (H_2O)_y$. Biochemically, they are defined as polyhydroxyaldehydes and polyhydroxyketones.

Carcinogenesis The production or origin of cancer.

Cardiac output The value calculated by multiplying the stroke volume by the heart rate.

Cardiomyopathy Refers to disease or disorder of the heart.

Caries Gradual decay of a bone, in particular, a tooth.

Carotenes Yellow pigments present in various plant and animal tissue, especially in yellow vegetables. Carotenes are precursor substances to vitamin A.

Catabolism Chemical reactions that are involved in the breaking down or fragmentation of molecules into smaller units.

Catalyst Substance that speeds up a chemical reaction without itself participating in the reaction.

Catecholamines Biochemically, refers to pyrocatechols with alkylamine side chains. Examples include epinephrine, norepinephrine, and dopamine.

Cation An ion with a positive charge.

Cellulose Fibrous carbohydrate substance found in the cell wall of plant cells. It serves as a supporting structure for plants.

Cheilosis Condition characterized by reddened lips and fissures at the angles. Results from a deficiency of riboflavin.

Chlorine Nonmetallic element belonging to the halogens. In the body it is found mainly combined with sodium and performs several physiological functions.

Cholesterol Lipid produced in the body that is used in the synthesis of several steroid hormones.

Cholicalciferol Form of vitamin D known as vitamin D_3 and produced within the body.

Choline Considered to be a nutritional factor in the B complex vitamin family. It is found in both plants and animals and is a component of lecithin and other phospholipids.

Chromium Metallic element that may have a physiological function in the body.

Chronotropic Pertains to an increase in heart rate.

Cirrhosis Liver disease characterized by tissue degeneration accompanied by fat and fiber infiltration.

Citrus bioflavonoids Also known as vitamin P. Substances thought to be necessary for the proper absorption of vitamin C in the body.

Coagulation The clotting of blood.

Cobalamin Vitamin B_{12}.

Cobalt Metallic element known to enhance erythropoiesis in animals.

Coenzyme An enzyme activator.

Cognition State of awareness, perception, and memory.

Colitis Inflammation of the colon.

Collagen Protein substance that exists in all tissues of the body.

Conjunctivitis Inflammation of the conjunctiva.

Copper Metallic element that plays an important physiological role in the body.

Corticosteroids Steroid hormones secreted by the adrenal cortex that play a role in metabolism.

Corticosterone An importnat corticosteroid produced by the adrenal gland that mainly functions in carbohydrate metabolism.

Cortisol Glucocorticoid secreted by the adrenal cortex. It is the main glucocorticoid in humans.

Cyanocobalamin Another name for vitamin B_{12}.

Cyclic AMP Cyclic 3′, 5′-adenosine monophosphate. It is a cyclic nucleotide that serves as an intracellular second messenger for many nonsteroid hormones.

Cystic fibrosis Of or pertaining to the formation of a cyst. Also, a disease involving the exocrine glands, particularly those that secrete mucous.

Cysteine Nonessential sulfur containing amino acid found among protein degradation products.

Cystine Obtained from the oxidation of cysteine and therefore a nonessential amino acid. It is also obtained from protein products.

Deficiency disorder Disease that occurs as a result of a lack of a substance in the body that is necessary for normal body metabolism.

Deoxyribonucleic acid   Nucleic acid found in all cells that stores and transmits genetic information. It consists of a double helix of nucleotide subunits.

Dermatitis   Inflammatory condition of the skin accompanied by redness, itching, and skin lesions.

Dessicated liver   Supplementary food that is a rich source of several of the vitamins and minerals.

Diabetes   Disorder characterized by higher than normal levels of glucose in the blood accompanied by the appearance of glucose in the urine as a result of an insulin deficiency.

Diastolic blood pressure   The pressure existing in the arteries during the relaxation phase between heartbeats. The normal value is approximately 80 mm Hg.

Diiodotyrosine   Substance formed during the chemical reactions taking place in the thyroid gland for the production of iodine.

Diuretic   Substance that causes an increase in urine production.

Diverticulosis   Inflammation of the diverticula of the colon. It can result in feces stagnation.

DNA   See deoxyribonucleic acid.

Dopamine   Neurotransmitter found in certain neural pathways of the brain.

Eczema   Inflammation of the cutaneous tissue. Considered to be more of a symptom than a disease.

Edema   Condition in which body tissues retain an excessive amount of tissue fluid. Can be generalized or local in nature.

Electrolyte   Substance that ionizes in solution. Some of the important electrolytes or ions in the body include Na^+, K^+, Cl^-, and HCO_3^-.

-emia   Suffix used to indicate factors relating to the blood. For example, hyponatremia refers to low levels of sodium in the blood.

Encephalopathy   Any dysfunction of the brain.

End-diastolic volume   The filling of the ventricles during diastole, which normally increases the volume of each ventricle to approximately 120 to 130 milliliters.

Endocrine   Glands that secrete hormones directly into the bloodstream.

Endogenous opiates Opiatelike substances that are produced directly within a cell or organism.

Enzymes Proteins that are synthesized by cells and that act as a catalyst in specific cellular reactions.

Epidemiology The study of epidemic diseases.

Epithelial cells Cells that line the outer surface of the body and line the body cavities. They also form the secreting portions of glands.

Ergocalciferol Form of vitamin D known as vitamin D_2. It is a synthetic substance and can be used as a therapeutic agent.

Ergosterol Substance used in the formation of vitamin D.

Essential amino acids Group of eight amino acids that are not manufactured by the body but are absolutely essential for life.

Estrogen The major female sex hormone, secreted by the ovary. It is responsible for the typical female characteristics.

Excitation-contraction coupling The process of nerve transmission coupled with muscle contraction.

Exercise The active functional processes of muscles.

Exocrine Glands that secrete their products directly into a duct or on a body surface.

Fats Also known as lipids. Fats are insoluble in water, and upon hydrolysis they break down into fatty acids and glycerol. They belong to the class of essential nutrients that supply energy to the body.

Fat-soluble Soluble in fats and not in water or aqueous solution. Fat-soluble substances generally are soluble in organic solvents such as ether, benzene, chloroform, and other fat solvents.

Fat-soluble vitamins Vitamins that are soluble only in fat solvents such as vitamins A, D, E, and K.

Ferritin Compound formed by combining the ferrous ion ($Fe++$) with a protein called apoferritin.

Fiber The indigestible part of foods, also referred to as roughage. It is composed of complex carbohydrates and is mainly derived from plants.

Fight or flight response Activation of the sympathetic-adrenal-medullary axis.

Fluorine   Nonmetallic element belonging to the group of halogens. It is essential for both plants and animals and appears to aid in the formation of bones and teeth.

Folacin   Another name for folic acid, a member of the B complex family of vitamins.

Folic acid   Member of the B complex family of vitamins. It is used in the treatment of anemia.

Follicle-stimulating hormone   Polypeptide hormone secreted by the anterior pituitary in both males and females. Also referred to as gonadotropin.

Free fatty acids   Compounds that are either saturated or unsaturated and are necessary for normal fat metabolism.

Gallium   Rare metallic substance found in bauxite.

***Gamma*-Aminobutyric acid**   Important neurotransmitter found in the brain.

Garlic   Herb that contains large amounts of vitamins B and C and some minerals.

General adaptation syndrome   Theoretical model used to describe the series of nervous and endocrine changes that take place during the experience of chronic stress.

Ginseng   Herb used medicinally in the Orient to alleviate weakness and fatigue.

Glucagon   Hormone secreted by the pancreas that influences blood sugar levels.

Glucocorticoid   Any of the steroid hormones secreted by the adrenal cortex that influence carbohydrate, fat, and protein metabolism.

Gluconeogenesis   The biochemical steps involved in the conversion of glucose from noncarbohydrate sources, such as proteins and fats.

Glucose   The simplest sugar found in the blood. It serves as the primary source of energy for cells.

Glutamic acid   Nonessential amino acid formed during the hydrolysis of proteins.

Glutamine   Nonessential amino acid.

Glycerol   Substance formed by the hydrolysis of fat.

Glycine Nonessential amino acid.

Glycogen Substance also known as animal starch. It is the form in which carbohydrates are stored in animals for future use.

Glycogenolysis The biochemical steps involving the conversion of glycogen into glucose.

Glycolysis Energy yielding conversion of glucose to lactic acid in several tissues of the body, particular that of muscle.

Gonadotropins Refers to the follicle-stimulating hormone (FSH) and luteinizing hormone (LH) secreted by the anterior pituitary gland.

Gout Metabolic disease characterized by inflammation of the joints and the large toe.

Growth Hormone Hormone released by the anterior pituitary gland that promotes the growth of the organism. It is also secreted during many types of stress exposure and is involved in nutrient metabolism.

Hair analysis Technique that provides a measure of the mineral content of the body. In particular, it is used to detect the presence of toxic mineral elements.

Halogen Substance that forms salts. One of a group of elements that exhibit similar properties.

HDL See high density lipoproteins.

Hemicellulose Form of plant fiber.

Hemoglobin Important blood protein, red, containing an iron pigment. It plays an important role in the transport of oxygen and carbon dioxide in the bloodstream.

Hemolysis Destruction of red blood cells occurring in such a manner as to liberate hemoglobin into the surrounding medium.

Hemophilia Hereditary blood disease characterized by a extremely prolonged coagulation time.

Hemosiderin Iron-containing protein whose source is hemoglobin.

Hemostasis The halting of blood loss. Also, stagnation of blood.

Heparin Substance that prevents blood coagulation.

Hepatic Pertaining to the liver.

High density lipoprotein Protein that binds cholesterol.

Histamine Substance found in the circulation wherever body tissue is traumatized or damaged.

Histidine Considered to be an essential amino acid in early childhood but nonessential in adults.

Homeostasis Equilibrium state with regard to the internal environment within the body with regard to the many functions and chemical composition of the tissues, fluids, and cells.

Hormone Substance produced by an endocrine gland that is secreted directly into the bloodstream.

5-Hydroxytryptamine Another name for serotonin.

Hyper- Prefix denoting excessiveness or above normal.

Hyperglycemia Blood sugar levels above normal.

Hypertension High blood pressure.

Hypertrophy Excessive enlargement of a tissue or organ.

Hypo- Prefix denoting deficiency or below normal.

Hypoglycemia Blood sugar levels below normal.

Hypoplasia Impaired development of a tissue.

Hypotension Low blood pressure.

Hypothalamus Important region of the brain in control of thirst and appetite , regulation of body temperature, metabolism, and secretion of endocrine glands.

Hypoxia Condition of lower than normal levels of oxygen present in the inspired air or in the blood or tissues.

Inositol Member of the vitamin B complex family.

Insulin Hormone secreted by the pancreas and essential for the maintenance of normal blood sugar levels and proper use of sugar by the body.

Iodine Nonmetallic element belonging to the halogen group of chemical elements. It is necessary for the proper functioning of the thyroid gland.

Iron Metallic element found abundantly in nature. It is necessary for life and forms an essential component of hemoglobin.

Ischemia Local obstruction of the circulation.

Isoleucine Essential amino acid.

Kaliuresis Refers to the excessive loss of potassium in the urine.

Kelp Substance found in seaweed that is a very rich source of several of the vitamins and minerals.

Keratinization Process of keratin formation. Keratin is a protein substance found in hair, nails, and other hard tissue.

Keratomalacia Condition resulting from a lack of vitamin A and characterized by a softening of the cornea.

Ketosis Condition of acidosis in the body characterized by the accumulation of ketone bodies such as acetone, acetoacetic acid, and beta-hydroxybutyric acid in the body.

Kwashiorkor Disease of malnutrition resulting from a protein deficiency in infancy or early childhood.

Lactate See lactic acid.

Lactation Secretion of milk in mammals.

Lactic acid Substance produced in muscle during activity as a result of glycogen breakdown or glycolysis.

Laetrile Another name for vitamin B_{17}.

LDL See low-density lipoprotein.

Lead Metallic element whose compounds are toxic.

Lecithin Fatty substance found in several tissues and belonging to a class of substances called phospholipids.

Legnin Form of plant fiber.

Leucine Essential amino acid.

Leucocyte The various types of white blood cells found in the blood.

Leukemia Disease characterized by an abnormal increase in leucocytes found in blood-forming organs. May be acute or chronic but is generally fatal.

Linoleic acid Unsaturated fatty acid.

Linolenic acid Unsaturated fatty acid.

Lipid See fats.

Lipolysis Process of fat breakdown or catabolism.

Lipoprotein Compound consisting of a protein and a lipid.

Lipophilic Substance that has an affinity for lipids.

Lithium Metallic element used in the treatment of mental disorders.

Low-density lipoprotein Protein that binds cholesterol.

Luteinizing hormone Polypeptide hormone secreted by the anterior pituitary gland that acts on the gonads. Also referred to as gonadotropin. In the male it is sometimes called interstitial cell-stimulating hormone.

Lymphocytopenia Decreased number of lymphocytes in the circulation.

Lysine Essential amino acid.

Macrocytic anemia Anemia characterized by red blood cells that are larger than normal in size.

Magnesium Metallic element found in the tissues of animals, particularly in muscle, bone, and extracellular fluids.

Manganese Metallic element found in many foods. It is also found in the cells of some plants and animals.

Mania Form of psychosis characterized by psychomotor overactivity.

Medulla Central or inner portion of an organ as distinct from the cortex, which forms the outer portion.

Megaloblastic anemia Anemia characterized by red blood cells larger than normal in size and nucleated.

Melanoma A usually malignant tumor containing melanin, a dark pigment.

Membrane permeabililty The ease by which ions and organic and inorganic molecules pass through a cell membrane.

Mercury Metallic element, liquid at room temperature, the salts of which are used medicinally as antiseptics.

Metabolic rate Also known as basal metabolic rate. The amount of energy the body needs for the maintenance of vital processes at rest.

Metabolism All the biochemical, physiological, and energy transformation changes that take place within an organism.

Metabolite Any of the several products of metabolism.

Methionine Essential amino acid.

Micro minerals See trace elements.

Mineral Inorganic element (or compound) found in nature. Several minerals are found in body tissue and perform vital physiological roles.

Mineralocorticoid Group of substances secreted by the adrenal cortex that are responsible for maintaining electrolyte balance in the body.

Molybdenum Metallic element present in many enzyme systems of the body.

Multiple Sclerosis Progressive disease of the central nervous system characterized by widespread areas of demyelinated glial tissue.

Muscle tone Normal tension as seen in response to various stimuli.

Muscular dystrophy Wasting away or atrophy of muscles.

Myodegeneration Degeneration of muscle tissue.

Myoglobin Pigment found in muscle that binds oxygen.

Myopathy Disease of striated muscle.

Na-K-ATPase Enzyme necessary for the active transport or the pumping of sodium and potassium ions across cell membranes.

Natriuresis Excessive loss of sodium in the urine.

Necrosis Tissue degeneration.

Nerve transmission Sending of information from one nerve to another through electrochemical impulses and neurotransmitter release.

Neuritis Inflammation of a nerve or nerves.

Neuroaxonal dystrophy Wasting away or atrophy of nerve tissue.

Neuroendocrine The combined activity of both the nervous and endocrine systems.

Neurosis Psychological disorder characterized primarily by anxiety.

Neurotransmitter Substance secreted at the axon endings of neurons that plays a role in impulse transmission across a synapse.

Niacin Member of the B complex family of vitamins.

Niacinamide Amide of niacin.

Nickel Metallic element whose salts are used for medicinal purposes.

Nicotinamide Amide of nicotinic acid.

Nicotinic acid Alternate name for niacin.

Nonessential amino acids Those amino acids that are produced within the body.

Norepinephrine Catecholamine produced by the adrenal medulla. It plays an important role in the stress response and is also a neurotransmitter in the brain and the autonomic nervous system.

Norleucine Nonessential amino acid.

Normotensive Normal blood pressure.

Nucleic acids Large molecules composed of nucleotides that form the basis of heredity and protein synthesis (see deoxyribonucleic acid and ribonucleic acid).

Nucleoprotein A combination of a protein and a nucleic acid. Nucleoproteins are found in the nuclei of all cells.

Nutrient Food substance necessary for normal body functioning.

Nutrition Process of supplying the body with the necessary nutrients to maintain normal physiological functioning.

Oleic Acid Oily, colorless liquid derived from fats. It is an unsaturated fatty acid whose salts are referred to as oleates.

Oncogenic Formation or production of tumors.

Orotic acid Alternate name for vitamin B_{13}.

Ornithine Amino acid that is an intermediate in the biosynthesis of urea.

Osteomalacia Disease characterized by a softening of the bones.

Osteoporosis Condition characterized by decrease in bone mass resulting in porous and fragile bones.

Oxidation Chemical combining of a substance with oxygen.

Oxygen consumption Grams of oxygen consumed per unit time during the course of cellular metabolism.

PABA See *para*-aminobenzoic acid.

Palmitic acid The most abundant fatty acid found in humans.

Pangamic acid Name given to vitamin B_{15}.

***Para*-Aminobenzoic acid** Member of the B complex family of vitamins.

Parasympathetic nervous system Craniosacral division of the autonomic nervous system.

Parathormone Another name given to parathyroid hormone.

Parathyroid hormone Hormone secreted by the parathyroid gland that regulates calcium levels in the blood.

Pectin Form of fibrous material.

Pellagra Deficiency disease resulting from a lack of the B vitamin niacin, characterized by gastrointestinal, neurological, and cutaneous symptoms.

Peripheral resistance The mean arterial pressure divided by the rate of blood flowing out of the heart per unit time. The resistance present in the systemic circulation that the blood flowing out of the heart must encounter.

Permeability See membrane permeability.

Permissive effect Refers to the necessary presence of one or more hormones to affect the specific physiological activity of another hormone.

Pernicious anemia Blood disease characterized by a graded decrease in red blood cells. It is accompanied by neurological disturbances and muscular weakness.

Peroxidation The combining of a substance with peroxides.

Phenylalanine Essential amino acid.

Phosphocreatine Substance found in muscle and composed of equal parts of phosphoric acid and creatine.

Phospholipids Substance consisting of phosphorus, fatty acids, and a nitrogenous base.

Phosphorus Nonmetallic element found only in the combined form. It is found in bone tissue principally combined with calcium.

Pituitary gland Gland composed of anterior, intermediate, and posterior portions, responsible for the secretion of several hormones in the body.

Polyribosomes Complex of ribosomal subunits assembled by messenger RNA and containing genetic information.

Polyunsaturated fats Fats that have many unsaturated bonds and that tend to be liquid at room temperature.

Potassium Metallic element that constitutes the principal element of intracellular fluids.

Progesterone Important female hormone secreted by the ovary. In particular, it plays an important role during pregnancy.

Prolactin Hormone secreted by the anterior pituitary gland that is involved in the process of lactation.

Proline Nonessential amino acid.

Prophylaxis The prevention of disease.

Proteins Nitrogenous substances necessary for life. When hydrolyzed, they produce amino acids.

Prothrombin Precursor to thrombin through its interaction with calcium salts in the circulation.

Provitamins Precursors of vitamins. These substances are normally inactive but under appropriate conditions can be converted into active vitamins.

Psoriasis Chronic inflammatory disease of the skin.

Psychophysiological The mental, emotional, and physiological aspects of an individual.

Pulmonary ventilation Refers to the inflow and outflow of air between the alveoli of the lungs and the atmosphere.

Pulse pressure Defined as the difference between the systolic and diastolic blood pressures.

Pyridoxine Alternate name for vitamin B_6.

Receptor Chemically, it refers to specific proteins either in plasma or in cells with which a chemical mediator combines to exert its physiological effects.

Recommended Daily Allowance Establisment of guidelines for the energy and nutrient needs of the body. In the United States, the RDAs indicate the quantity of nutrients and calories necessary to nourish people who are healthy. They are by no means a standard for minimum requirements.

Releasing factors See releasing hormones.

Releasing hormones Hormones secreted by the hypothalamus that stimulate the anterior pituitary gland to secrete its hormones.

Renin-angiotensin Renin is a protein hormone that acts in the capacity of an enzyme, converting a blood globulin into the hormone angiotensin, a powerful vasoconstrictor.

Retinol Name given to vitamin A.

Rheumatic fever Systemic inflammatory disorder frequently followed by serious heart disease.

Riboflavin Name given to vitamin B_2.

Ribonucleic acid Nucleic acid involved in genetic information decoding. It exists in three forms, messenger RNA, ribosomal RNA, and transfer RNA.

Rickets Disease resulting from a vitamin D deficiency and characterized by osteomalacia.

RNA See ribonucleic acid.

Rose hips Seeds found in roses that are rich in vitamin C.

Rutin Related to hesperidin. It is used to restore increased fragility of the capillaries back to normal.

Saturated fats Fats containing only saturated bonds and no unsaturated linkages. These substances are saturated because they cannot accept more hydrogen linkages.

Schizophrenia Psychotic disorder characterized by withdrawal from objective reality and disintegration of personality, accompanied by hallucinations and delusions.

Selenium Metallic element chemically similar to sulfur and having wide industrial uses.

Serine Nonessential amino acid.

Serotonin Substance that is a neurotransmitter of the central nervous system. It also plays a role in several physiological functions in the body.

Silicon Nonmetallic element existing abundantly in nature.

Silicosis Occupational disease caused by inhaling dust containing silica. It is developed over a period of many years and is characterized by progressive fibrosis of the lungs.

Silver Metallic element whose salts are used medicinally for their antiseptic properties.

Skeletal muscle Composed of multinucleated, elongated, and transversely striated muscle fibers.

Sodium Metallic element that constitutes the principle cation of extracellular fluids.

Somatomedin Substance capable of stimulating certain anabolic processes in bone and cartilage and dependent on the activity of growth hormone.

Spirulina High-protein food rich in many of the vitamins and minerals.

Splanchnic Referring to the viscera.

Sprue Disease characterized by weakness and weight loss, often accompanied by various digestive disturbances.

Stearic acid Fatty acid found abundantly in animals and used in many pharmacological preparations.

Sterol Organic substances composed of 27 or more carbon atoms with one OH group (alcohol). An abundant sterol in animals is cholesterol.

Stimulus Anything in either the internal or external environment that can elicit a response in a muscle, gland, or nerve and that can accelerate metabolic processes in the body.

Stress Changes that occur in the body as a result of the organism's perception of a stimulus as a threat, whether mental, emotional, or physical or a combination of these factors.

Stress response The many biochemical, physiological, and behavioral changes taking place in the body as a result of the experience of stress.

Stroke volume Volume of blood ejected from the heart per beat.

Strontium Metallic element belonging to the group of alkaline earth elements. It is chemically similar to calcium.

Sulfur Element that combines with both metals and nonmetals to form sulfides. It is used medicinally to treat rheumatism, gout, skin disease, and other disorders.

Sympathetic nervous system Thoracic lumbar division of the autonomic nervous system. It is activated during the elicitation of the stress response.

Systolic pressure Pressure developed in the arteries as a result of the force exerted by the contraction of the left ventricle of the heart.

Tachycardia Rapid hearbeat, usually over 100 beats per minute.

Tension State of being stretched or strained.

Testosterone Major male sex hormone secreted by the testes. It is responsible for the typical male characteristics.

Thiamine Another name for vitamin B_1.

Thiazide Substance used as a diuretic.

Threonine Essential amino acid.

Thiouracil Antithyroid drug that inhibits the synthesis of thyroid hormones. It produces hypothyroidism.

Thrombin Enzyme in blood that converts fibrinogen into fibrin.

Thymicolymphatic atrophy Atrophy or involution of the lymphatic tissue of the thymus gland.

Thyrocalcitonin Hormone secreted by the thyroid gland that plays a role in regulating the levels of calcium in the blood. Also known as calcitonin.

Thyroid hormones The major hormones secreted by the thyroid gland, thyroxine and triiodothyronine.

Thyroxine Major hormone secreted by the thyroid gland.

Tidal volume During quiet breathing, the volume of air that is inhaled during inspiration and exits the lungs passively during expiration.

Tin Metallic element that is used in medicine.

Titanium Metallic element found in the combined form in minerals.

Tocopherols Group of different compounds that have vitamin E-like activity.

Tocotrinols Group of substances that have vitamin E-like activity and are similar in structure to the tocopherols.

Toxic Pertaining to substances that are poisonous to the body.

Trace elements Minerals normally found in minute amounts in food and tissues.

Triglyceride Substance composed of three molecules of fatty acids esterified to glycerol. It is a neutral fat and, upon hydrolysis, releases free fatty acids into the circulation.

Triiodothyronine Important hormone secreted by the thyroid gland.

Tryptophan Essential amino acid.

Tyrosine Nonessential amino acid.

Uric acid Organic acid that is the end-product of purine metabolism in the body.

Uricemia Excess uric acid in the blood.

Valine Essential amino acid.

Vanadium Metallic element widely found in nature, especially in phosphate sources.

Vasoconstriction Constriction of blood vessels.

Vasodilation Dilation or a widening of blood vessels.

Venous return Amount of blood that returns to the heart through the venous system.

Ventricular volume Volume of blood found in the ventricle. This amount varies depending on the phase of the cardiac cycle.

Very low-density lipoprotein Protein that binds cholesterol.

Vitamins Organic substances existing in most foods that are necessary for life, and the absence of which results in malnutrition or a specific deficiency disorder.

Vitamin F Formally used term for the essential fatty acids.

Vitamin G Obsolete term for vitamin B_2 or riboflavin.

Vitamin H Name formerly given to biotin (see biotin).

Vitamin H[1] Alternate name for *para*-aminobenzoic acid.

Vitamin L Substance thought to be necessary for lactation in rats.

Vitamin M Obsolete name for folic acid, a member of the vitamin B complex vitamin family.

Vitamin P Substances associated with vitamin C, including the citrus bioflavonoids, hesperidin, and rutin.

Vitamin P-P Alternate name for niacinamide, a member of the vitamin B complex family.

Vitamin T Substance that may play a role in blood coagulaton.

Vitamin U Substance that may protect against ulcer formation.

VLDL See very low-density lipoprotein.

Water-soluble vitamins Vitamins soluble only in aqueous solution, such as the B complex vitamins and vitamin C.

Waxes Form of plant fiber.

Wheat germ Kernal part of the wheat, a rich source of protein and several vitamins and minerals.

Xerophthalmia   Disease caused by a vitamin A deficiency and characterized by dryness of the conjunctiva.

Xerosis   Condition of abnormal dryness of the skin.

Yeast   Supplementary food that is a rich source of the vitamins, minerals, and protein.

Zinc   Metallic element that plays an important role in many enzymatic reactions of the body.

INDEX

ABOUT THE AUTHOR

Mary F. Asterita, Ph.D., is on the faculty at the Indiana University School of Medicine. She is also a lecturer at Purdue University and past president of the Biofeedback Society of Illinois. She is presently Director of Clinical Services and President of Biofeedback and Stress Management Services. Dr. Asterita has presented lectures, seminars, and workshops in the field of stress physiology and biofeedback for health care groups, business and industry, and other professional groups throughout the country and abroad. She is the author of *The Physiology of Stress: With Special Reference to the Neuroendocrine System.*

Dr. Asterita received her M.S. in physics from New York University, her Ph.D. in physiology from Cornell University, and her postdoctoral training at the Yale University School of Medicine.